THE
✚DANIEL
PLAN
JOURNAL

FAITH + FOOD + FITNESS + FOCUS + FRIENDS

THE
+DANIEL
PLAN
JOURNAL

40 DAYS *to a* HEALTHIER LIFE

RICK WARREN
& THE DANIEL PLAN TEAM

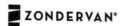

ZONDERVAN

The Daniel Plan Journal
Copyright © 2013 by The Daniel Plan

This title is also available as a Zondervan ebook. Visit www.zondervan.com/ebooks.

Requests for information should be addressed to:

Zondervan, Grand Rapids, Michigan 49530

ISBN 978-0-310-34432-2

Cover design: Curt Diepenhorst
Interior design: Sarah Johnson
Interior production: Beth Shagene
Editors: Andrea Vinley Jewell and Jim Ruark

Printed in the United States of America

13 14 15 16 17 18 /DCI/ 20 19 18 17 16 15 14 13 12 11 10 9 8 7 6 5 4 3 2 1

Contents

Bible Versions

MEDICAL DISCLAIMER

Welcome to a
New Way of Life

Even though I grew up in the church, I have never heard a single sermon about the body. Not one. I have heard sermons about the importance of your spirit, your soul, your mind, your character, and your values.

I believe it's safe to say most Christians don't have a "theology of health." Yet the Bible teaches us that our bodies are very important to God, and he wants us to take care of them.

We developed the biblically based Daniel Plan at Saddleback to help you understand what God says about your body and why it's important physically, mentally, and spiritually to maintain good health. God created you with a purpose. To fulfill that purpose, you need to take care of the body God gave you. Doing so will give you more energy. It will increase your stamina. It will help you handle stress and maintain a positive attitude.

We have designed this journal to guide and encourage you through the first forty days of The Daniel Plan. Every day we will provide you with biblical inspiration that teaches the spiritual significance of getting healthy and staying healthy, while reminding you that God is for you and your success in The Daniel Plan.

In addition, we will give you a tip or short activity to help you take one step at a time toward your health goals. We will also ask you questions so you can assess your health, stay motivated, track your progress, and adopt new habits.

Describing your journey in a written format helps you to stay focused on your goals and provides you with a motivational record that ultimately helps to sustain your momentum. Making progress in one area often spills over and creates a positive impact in other areas. This progress develops a win-win cycle to keep you moving forward.

Most of all, we hope The Daniel Plan will help you stay focused on God. As you depend on him more and more, you will become stronger. And instead of craving other things that don't support your goals, you will crave your time alone with him.

I have been a pastor for more than thirty-five years, and I have noticed that there tends to be three major reasons we give up on our many commitments to get and stay healthy:

1. We try to change through willpower instead of God's power. For most of us, willpower will work for about three weeks. Then we get tired and frustrated and go back to activities that are harmful to our health. By its very nature, willpower means you are forcing yourself to do something your body doesn't want you to do. That is why most of our New Year's resolutions don't last. We try to keep them by willpower instead of God power.

2. We try to change using wrong motivations instead of God motivations. When the goal is all about "me" — how

I look or feel — it's usually not enough to keep most people going. There's nothing wrong with those types of goals. In fact, looking healthy and feeling healthy are good goals.

But we need something greater than ourselves to help us stick it out, particularly when the journey gets tough. The Daniel Plan lifestyle supports your health and maximizes your ability to fulfill the mission God has planned for you.

3. We try to change by ourselves instead of with other people. You were made to grow and mature in community. It's nearly impossible to have lasting change in your life without support and encouragement from others. That's why we emphasize the need for friends as you work toward better health.

Going through The Daniel Plan with others weaves pleasure into your journey. That doesn't mean it will be easy, but it does mean you will have the joy of knowing you are accepted and loved by friends who are as committed to good health as you are.

I believe you will enjoy life on The Daniel Plan. Most people find their energy increases, they start sleeping better, their relationship with Christ deepens, and their whole outlook on life becomes brighter. Their motivation kicks up a notch, and the benefits start rolling in. I can't wait to hear how God will use a healthier you in the years to come. Welcome to an amazing, lifelong journey!

How to Use This Journal

Now you have a better picture of what The Daniel Plan is all about, and we hope you are eager to get started. Establishing a habit of journaling is going to support everything you do to move forward into better health. It doesn't matter if you are an avid journal writer or you are trying it for the first time. We have made it easy by creating a daily template to track your progress over the next forty days. In fact, we think you will enjoy the benefits of journaling so much that you may want to continue well past your first forty days!

You will begin each day with a biblically based Daily Reflection to which you can personally respond, creating a faith-centered approach to your experience. This is what makes our journal unique: Faith is the starting point.

Then you will explore your progress in each of the other Essentials (Food, Fitness, Focus, and Friends) by answering the questions in the Daily Check-In. It's important to track how you are doing in all Essentials. You may feel that you have a better handle on one or two, but challenge yourself by exploring each one and being honest about where you need to focus your efforts.

Part of your Daily Check-In examines what you eat, which

is vital to achieving better health. Soon you will discover patterns related to your eating habits that will clarify much of the "why" behind your choices. You will also record how much water you are drinking. Hydration is key, because often when you think you are hungry, you are just dehydrated!

With this journal, you will quickly realize that keeping yourself accountable is directly tied to your success. We hope this journal offers you much more than just pages to record your progress; in fact it is our prayer that you will move into a deeper relationship with God.

Before You Start

Take a few days to set goals, review The Daniel Plan food guidelines, assess where you are with each of the five Essentials, and record your current state of health. Proverbs 4:26 says, "Give careful thought to the paths for your feet and be steadfast in all your ways."

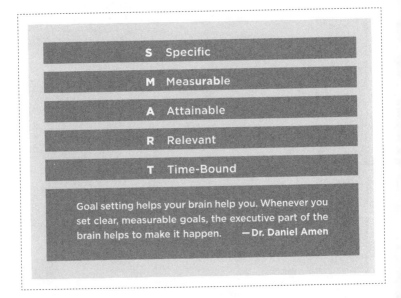

S	Specific
M	Measurable
A	Attainable
R	Relevant
T	Time-Bound

Goal setting helps your brain help you. Whenever you set clear, measurable goals, the executive part of the brain helps to make it happen. **—Dr. Daniel Amen**

SMART
GOALS

Set SMART (Specific, Measurable, Attainable, Relevant, and Time-bound) Goals, similar to what we talked about in chapter 6 in *The Daniel Plan* on the Focus Essential. Goal setting is a spiritual discipline like prayer and spending time alone with God. In fact, goals can be an act of stewardship or worship where you say, "God, I want to make the most of what I've been given" or "God, I give you back the life you've given to me, and I want to go in your direction."

Specific goals are clear and distinct. This is where you understand exactly what is expected and why it is important. A specific goal usually answers the five "W" questions:

- What?
- Why?
- Who?
- Where?
- Which? (Identify the requirements and constraints in the areas of faith, food, fitness, focus, and friends.)

To set specific goals, you need to know the difference between pressures and priorities, activity and achievement, and what's urgent and what's important. If you focus your energy on goals that aren't God-directed, your energy won't have much power. Paul modeled this in 1 Corinthians 9:26: "Therefore I do not run like someone running aimlessly; I do not fight like a boxer beating the air." Energy that is focused has enormous power.

Measurable emphasizes the need for tangible benchmarks. If a goal is not measurable, how will you know whether you are making progress? Measuring your progress helps you stay on track and keeps you excited. A measurable goal answers questions such as "How much?" and "By when?"

Attainable means the goals need to be realistic, even though it's okay to have big dreams. Extreme goals usually invite failure and frustration. When you identify the goals that are most important to you, you will figure out ways to make them happen.

At the same time, you also need to realize that attainable doesn't mean only the goals you can accomplish in your own power. If you can do it in your own power, then you don't really need any faith. Goals can stretch your faith and affirm your trust in God.

Relevant means goals that matter. A relevant goal answers "yes" to these questions: Is it worthwhile? Is this the right time? Does it match your other efforts and needs?

This also means your goals are relevant to God and bring him glory. Any goal that brings you closer to God and makes you want to serve him and others is a goal that matters. The apostle Paul encouraged us to "make it our goal to please him, whether we are at home in the body or away from it" (2 Corinthians 5:9).

Time-bound stresses the importance of attaining the goal within a certain time frame. When you use time-bound criteria, you will be able to measure your goals and focus your efforts on a specific deadline.

Here are examples of seven SMART Goals:

1. Lose 30 pounds in six months.

2. Walk, as if I am late, four times a week for forty-five minutes with my walking partner.

3. Do a complete kitchen cleanse (that is, clean out the kitchen of all unhealthful food) once a week.

4. Spend one night a week with friends reading and discussing The Daniel Plan material. Call in between meetings for encouragement and accountability.

5. Spend five to ten minutes a day journaling my progress.

6. Spend ten or more minutes a day in prayer or reading my Bible.

7. Eat Daniel Plan – approved foods at least 90 percent of the time.

Working toward SMART Goals will give you the direction you need to focus on what's really important. You will record these on pages 22 – 24 and revisit them every ten days.

THE DANIEL PLAN
PLATE

Over the next forty days you will be tracking your food. That is why we created The Daniel Plan plate. Following the plate as closely as you can will keep you focused on foods that truly love you back! As you learn to use the plate guidelines, you will maximize your energy, kick-start your metabolism, and curb your cravings. Don't worry, we know that every day is *not* perfect. In fact, The Daniel Plan journey is all about progress, *not* perfection. It's about taking steps in the right direction.

Goals are like magnets that pull you forward when you feel like giving up. They give you hope!

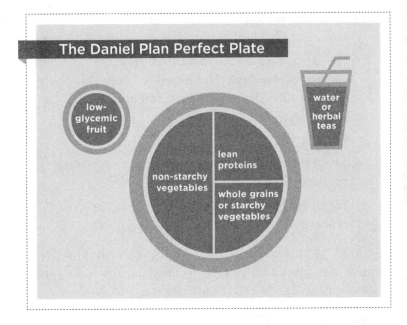

The Daniel Plan gives an easy guideline to use for any meal:

- 50% non-starchy veggies
- 25% healthy animal or vegetable proteins
- 25% healthy starch or whole grains
- Side of low-glycemic fruit
- Drink — water or herbal iced teas

Here are some great choices to start with. For more ideas, be sure to visit *danielplan.com* or download The Daniel Plan App for delicious recipes and more.

NON-STARCHY VEGGIES	PROTEIN	STARCH OR GRAIN	LOW-GLYCEMIC FRUIT
Asparagus	Beans	Beets	Apples
Bell peppers	Beef	Brown/Black Rice	Blackberries
Broccoli	Chicken	Carrots	Blueberries
Cauliflower	Eggs	Buckwheat	Gogi berries
Collard greens	Halibut	Green Peas	Grapefruit
Cucumbers	Lentils	Corn	Plums
Green beans	Nuts	Quinoa	Kiwi
Kale	Salmon	Sweet potatoes	Nectarines
Spinach	Seeds	Turnips	Peaches
Zucchini	Turkey	Winter Squash	Raspberries

THE DANIEL PLAN 5
ESSENTIALS SURVEY

It is very important to remember that we all have different starting points. It's a great idea to assess your health in each of the five Essentials before you start and at the completion of the program. On a scale of 1 – 5, please rate your current status for each of The Daniel Plan Essentials. We would encourage you to take this survey before your program begins and after it ends.

FAITH	Very Dissatisfied	Dissatisfied	Neutral	Satisfied	Very Satisfied
1. Relationship with God	1	2	3	4	5
2. Sense of meaning and purpose *in life*	1	2	3	4	5
3. Spiritual practices: prayer, worship, meditation	1	2	3	4	5
4. Spiritual growth	1	2	3	4	5
5. Giving to others	1	2	3	4	5

Add up each column and enter your total Faith Score: _____

FOOD	Never	Rarely	Sometimes	Most of the time	Daily
1. I eat 7 or more servings of a variety of vegetables and fruits.	1	2	3	4	5
2. I eat lean protein with every meal.	1	2	3	4	5
3. I drink 8 to 10 glasses of water every day.	1	2	3	4	5
4. I choose healthy fats.	1	2	3	4	5
5. I eat a healthy, nutritious breakfast.	1	2	3	4	5

Add up each column and enter your total Food Score: _____

FITNESS	Very Dissatisfied	Dissatisfied	Neutral	Satisfied	Very Satisfied
1. My body (appearance/ weight)	1	2	3	4	5
2. My cardiovascular endurance	1	2	3	4	5
3. My strength	1	2	3	4	5
4. My flexibility	1	2	3	4	5
5. My physical health	1	2	3	4	5

Add up each column and enter your total Fitness Score: _____

FOCUS	Very Dissatisfied	Dissatisfied	Neutral	Satisfied	Very Satisfied
1. Positive mental attitude	1	2	3	4	5
2. Achievement of personal goals	1	2	3	4	5
3. Peace of mind	1	2	3	4	5
4. Gratitude and thankfulness	1	2	3	4	5
5. Ability to handle mistakes or failures	1	2	3	4	5

Add up each column and enter your total Focus Score: _____

FRIENDS	Very Dissatisfied	Dissatisfied	Neutral	Satisfied	Very Satisfied
1. Relationship with my significant other	1	2	3	4	5
2. Relationships with my family	1	2	3	4	5
3. Relationships with my friends	1	2	3	4	5
4. Relationships with others (co-workers or neighbors)	1	2	3	4	5
5. My communication skills	1	2	3	4	5

Add up each column and enter your total Friends Score: _____

DANIEL PLAN ESSENTIALS
SURVEY RESULTS

Congratulations! Now that you have completed your survey, transfer your scores for each area of wellness (Faith, Food, Fitness, Focus, and Friends) into the following table in the "My Score" column. Then read the following pages to get a better understanding of what your scores mean and figure out what areas you need to focus on most. Be sure to log onto The Daniel Plan website at *danielplan.com* to learn about the Stages of Change and how to move forward with your program.

	MY SCORE
FAITH	
FOOD	
FITNESS	
FOCUS	
FRIENDS	

YOUR SCORE:

Score of 20–25: Well done! If you scored between 20 and 25 points for a particular Daniel Plan Essential, your answers demonstrate that you are aware of the importance of this area to your personal wellness and have developed the habits to rate it so highly.

Score of 15–20: If you scored between 15 and 20 in one or more of The Daniel Plan Essentials, your health and wellness practices are doing well, but you may have room for some improvement. Identify the areas you are dissatisfied with and begin to review tips and strategies in *The Daniel Plan, The Daniel Plan* DVD Study and Study Guide, and companion tools to help improve your score the next time you take this survey.

Score of 10–15: If you scored between 10 and 15 in one or more of The Daniel Plan Essentials, this may be an ideal area to focus your attention on and set specific goals.

Scores below 5–10: If you scored below a 10 in one or more of The Daniel Plan Essentials, it is time to make some changes. Identify all of the areas where you scored yourself with a 1 or a 2 and consider improving these items.

Now that you have your scores in hand, you may want to focus on one or two Essentials, or maybe all five. Remember this is *your* journey. We all have different starting points, so stay focused on what you want to achieve. It's great to check in with friends to get ideas, but don't get sidetracked by comparing yourself to others. What's most important is that *you* are taking small steps in the right direction.

40-Day Health Assessment

	DAY 1
Height	
Weight	
BMI*	
Blood Pressure	
Waist	
Hips	
Activity Level**	

*Refer to page 199 to calculate your BMI.
****Sedentary** (I rarely or never do any physical activities)
Light (I do some light or moderate physical activities every week)
Regular (I do moderate physical activities every week, 20–30 minutes a day for 3–4 days a week)
Active to vigorous (I do moderate to vigorous physical activities every week, 30–60 minutes a day for 5 or more days a week)

You can also track your health assessment online (*danielplan.com*) or with The Daniel Plan App.

SET SMART GOALS
FOR THE NEXT 40 DAYS

Choose one or two Essentials to focus on, and reassess your SMART Goals as you go.

- **FAITH:**
  (Example: "Start my day by reading the Bible.")

- **FOOD:**
  ("Clean out my pantry of all unhealthful food.")

- **FITNESS:**
  ("Walk as if I'm late four to five times a week.")

- **FOCUS:**
  ("Eat Daniel Plan – approved foods at least 90 percent of the time.")

- **FRIENDS:**
  ("Find friends who want to go on this journey with me.")

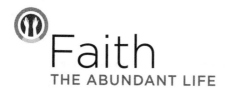

Faith
THE ABUNDANT LIFE

Jesus [said], "... I came so they can have real and eternal life, more and better life than they ever dreamed of."
— John 10:10 MSG

DAILY
REFLECTION

Jesus wants you to experience the fullness of life. Your relationship with him enables you to pack meaning and purpose into each and every moment. Jesus says this abundant life in him will be better than all your dreams rolled into one.

In this real and eternal life, every part of you is interconnected: your spiritual health is connected to your physical health, and they are both connected to your mental and emotional health. A problem in one area will affect all the others.

God shaped you with this interconnectedness, so on your journey you must learn to trust that he has also given you the means and methods to maintain the good health necessary for an abundant life. God never intended for you to sit on the sidelines, unable to stay engaged in the fullness of life. He wants you to move forward toward greater energy and productivity with eternal significance.

What are the resources and means already in your life that will help you achieve your goals in The Daniel Plan?

How would your life be fuller if you were able to reach your health goals? What will you be able to do and accomplish with greater energy and better health?

FAITH

- How has your health hindered you from participating in the life God has for you?

DAILY
CHECK-IN

FOOD

- How did your meals align with The Daniel Plan plate today?

- How would you rate your eating today on a scale of 1 to 10 (10 being best):

| 1 | 2 | 3 | 4 | 5 | 6 | 7 | 8 | 9 | 10 |

- Some of the best choices I made today were:
  (e.g., eating a healthy breakfast)

👟 FITNESS

- What type of fitness/movement did you do today?

- Duration:

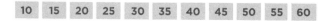

💡 FOCUS

- Gratitude for today:

- Goal for tomorrow:

👥 FRIENDS

- Who encouraged, supported, or joined you on your health journey today?

- Who needs your encouragement, support, or companionship?

DAILY
FOOD TRACKER

- What did you eat? How did it make you feel?

  BREAKFAST:

  SNACK:

  LUNCH:

  SNACK:

  DINNER:

  WATER: HOW MUCH WATER DID YOU DRINK?

- When you ate today, was it because you were hungry? Or were you motivated by boredom, stress, or fatigue?

- What worked?

- Any adjustments or changes for tomorrow?

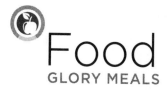

Food
GLORY MEALS

So whether you eat or drink or whatever you do, do it all for the glory of God.

— *1 Corinthians 10:31*

DAILY
REFLECTION

Food is a gift from God, and it is meant to be savored. When you hurry through meals, you tend to overeat, and you miss the point of the gift. Slow down and appreciate the tastes, textures, and pleasures that good food can give. Today, instead of eating in your car or standing at the sink, try sitting down for each meal and taking your time.

> "If you want to form a new habit, get to work, if you want to break a bad habit, get on your knees."
>
> —Marie T. Freeman

Meals are moments when you can refocus on God and thank him for providing you with the food you eat. It's also a time when you can connect with friends and enjoy a meal together, celebrating what God is doing in your lives.

What might happen to the way you experience food if you simply slow down and take time to appreciate each bite as well as the company with whom you eat?

🎭 FAITH

- One of the ways we eat to the glory of God is by choosing foods that are good for our bodies. God gave these foods to us to keep us healthy. How does knowing this help you decide what to eat?

DAILY
CHECK-IN

🌀 FOOD

- How did your meals align with The Daniel Plan plate today?

- How would you rate your eating today on a scale of 1 to 10 (10 being best):

| 1 | 2 | 3 | 4 | 5 | 6 | 7 | 8 | 9 | 10 |

- Some of the best choices I made today were:
  (e.g., eating a healthy breakfast)

🏃 FITNESS

- What type of fitness/movement did you do today?

- Duration:

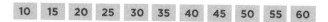

💡 FOCUS

- Gratitude for today:

- Goal for tomorrow:

👥 FRIENDS

- Who encouraged, supported, or joined you on your health journey today?

- Who needs your encouragement, support, or companionship?

DAILY
FOOD TRACKER

- What did you eat? How did it make you feel?

  BREAKFAST:

  SNACK:

  LUNCH:

  SNACK:

  DINNER:

  WATER: HOW MUCH WATER DID YOU DRINK?

- When you ate today, was it because you were hungry?
  Or were you motivated by boredom, stress, or fatigue?

- What worked?

- Any adjustments or changes for tomorrow?

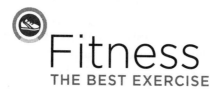

Fitness
THE BEST EXERCISE

The LORD is my strength and my shield....
My heart leaps for joy, and with my song I praise him.
— Psalm 28:7

DAILY
REFLECTION

Think about this: God would not have designed your body to need physical exercise and at the same time make exercise the most grueling, tedious thing you have to do.

God knows we are all shaped differently, so there's an "exercise" out there for every one of us. The best exercise is the one that you will actually do because you enjoy it. So what do you love? What sounds like fun? Ask God to show you what it is, and give it a try, even if it takes you out of your comfort zone.

Here's a good place to start: Move toward joy. If you think of exercise as drudgery, as an *ought to* in your life, your motivation

> Joy is part of the fruit of the Spirit (Galatians 5:22). Often I am inclined to think that joy is the motor, the thing that keeps everything else going.
>
> —Richard Foster,
> *Celebration of Discipline*

will disappear. If you direct your energies wisely and do something you enjoy, something you *get to do*, you will find that motivation comes naturally.

Today, journal about a time you had fun engaging in physical activity — as an adult and as a kid. What activities do you enjoy or did you once enjoy before you got too busy?

ⓝ FAITH

- Now write down "Move toward joy," and write what comes to mind when you reflect on that sentence. Then pick one activity and go do it!

DAILY
CHECK-IN

ⓕ FOOD

- How did your meals align with The Daniel Plan plate today?

- How would you rate your eating today on a scale of 1 to 10 (10 being best):

| 1 | 2 | 3 | 4 | 5 | 6 | 7 | 8 | 9 | 10 |

- Some of the best choices I made today were:
  (e.g., eating a healthy breakfast)

🏃 FITNESS

- What type of fitness/movement did you do today?

- Duration:

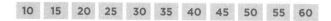

💡 FOCUS

- Gratitude for today:

- Goal for tomorrow:

👥 FRIENDS

- Who encouraged, supported, or joined you on your health journey today?

- Who needs your encouragement, support, or companionship?

DAILY
FOOD TRACKER

- What did you eat? How did it make you feel?

  BREAKFAST:

  SNACK:

  LUNCH:

  SNACK:

  DINNER:

  WATER: HOW MUCH WATER DID YOU DRINK?

- When you ate today, was it because you were hungry?
  Or were you motivated by boredom, stress, or fatigue?

- What worked?

- Any adjustments or changes for tomorrow?

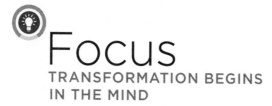

Focus
TRANSFORMATION BEGINS IN THE MIND

*Do not conform to the pattern of this world,
but be transformed by the renewing of your mind.*
— Romans 12:2

DAILY
REFLECTION

You may think transformation of your health begins with physical effort, but the truth is, if you want lasting change in your life, you need to refocus your mind.

When you trade your old thinking for new thinking, that's when transformation starts to happen. Ephesians 4:24 says, "Put on the new self, created to be like God in true righteousness and holiness."

To renew your mind, you're going to have to let go of the old attitudes, the old thought patterns, the old images that you have been living with so you can put on the new garments God has for you.

🧑 FAITH

- Which of your thought patterns may be unhealthy or untrue? Ask God to transform your mind with his truth.

- Dr. Amen wrote a book called *Change Your Brain, Change Your Life*. How do you do that? What are you feeding your brain that needs to be replaced with truth?

- Whatever you focus on is what you move toward. Spend some time writing down the things that you want in your life and praying that God will change your focus so you can move forward.

DAILY
CHECK-IN

🍎 FOOD

- How did your meals align with The Daniel Plan plate today?

- How would you rate your eating today on a scale of 1 to 10 (10 being best):

  1 2 3 4 5 6 7 8 9 10

- Some of the best choices I made today were:
  (*e.g., eating a healthy breakfast*)

🏃 FITNESS

- What type of fitness/movement did you do today?

- Duration:

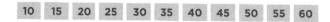

10 15 20 25 30 35 40 45 50 55 60

💡 FOCUS

- Gratitude for today:

- Goal for tomorrow:

👥 FRIENDS

- Who encouraged, supported, or joined you on your
  health journey today?

- Who needs your encouragement, support, or
  companionship?

DAILY
FOOD TRACKER

- What did you eat? How did it make you feel?

  BREAKFAST:

  SNACK:

  LUNCH:

  SNACK:

  DINNER:

  WATER: HOW MUCH WATER DID YOU DRINK?

- When you ate today, was it because you were hungry? Or were you motivated by boredom, stress, or fatigue?

- What worked?

- Any adjustments or changes for tomorrow?

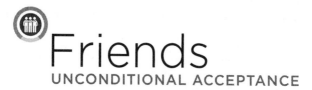

Friends
UNCONDITIONAL ACCEPTANCE

Accept one another, then, just as Christ accepted you,
in order to bring praise to God.

— Romans 15:7

DAILY
REFLECTION

God accepts us despite our messy lives, impure motives, and irritating attitudes (Ephesians 1:6). One of the ways we reflect God's love and bring him glory is to accept each other just as he accepts us. This means we accept others' quirks and look past their faults in order to see a person created in the image of God.

This acceptance makes your friends feel safe with you. This acceptance is what you need for support on The Daniel Plan. To have that kind of critical support with your friends, you will need to accept one another unconditionally.

This acceptance creates a safe environment where people are not afraid to express their fears and doubts or talk about their struggles and where lasting change starts.

Why do you think people are more likely to change after, rather than before, they find acceptance? How can you reach out with acceptance to a friend or person in your Daniel Plan group?

FAITH

- Either within this journal or on a piece of paper you plan to throw away, write down five events from your past that make it hard for you to believe God accepts you.

DAILY
CHECK-IN

FOOD

- How did your meals align with The Daniel Plan plate today?

- How would you rate your eating today on a scale of 1 to 10 (10 being best):

| 1 | 2 | 3 | 4 | 5 | 6 | 7 | 8 | 9 | 10 |

- Some of the best choices I made today were:
  (*e.g., eating a healthy breakfast*)

🟢 FITNESS

- What type of fitness/movement did you do today?

- Duration:

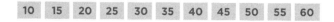

| 10 | 15 | 20 | 25 | 30 | 35 | 40 | 45 | 50 | 55 | 60 |

🔵 FOCUS

- Gratitude for today:

- Goal for tomorrow:

🟢 FRIENDS

- Who encouraged, supported, or joined you on your
  health journey today?

- Who needs your encouragement, support, or
  companionship?

DAILY
FOOD TRACKER

- What did you eat? How did it make you feel?

  BREAKFAST:

  SNACK:

  LUNCH:

  SNACK:

  DINNER:

  WATER: HOW MUCH WATER DID YOU DRINK?

- When you ate today, was it because you were hungry?
  Or were you motivated by boredom, stress, or fatigue?

- What worked?

- Any adjustments or changes for tomorrow?

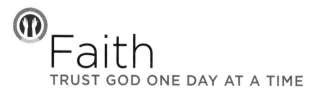

Faith
TRUST GOD ONE DAY AT A TIME

"Give us today our daily bread."
— Matthew 6:11

DAILY
REFLECTION

Notice the Bible doesn't say, "Give us today our *weekly* bread" or "Give us today our *yearly* bread."

God wants you to trust him one day at a time. You don't need to be concerned about tomorrow until tomorrow. You don't need to be concerned about next week until next week.

This means you don't have to stress about all the future steps necessary to make you *Daniel Strong*. You just need to focus on what you need to do for today. You can focus on succeeding at The Daniel Plan one day at a time.

Jesus said, "So don't worry about tomorrow, for tomorrow will bring its own worries. Today's trouble is enough for today" (Matthew 6:34 NLT).

FAITH

- Why do you think God wants you to take it one day at a time?

- Make a list of all your concerns related to your Daniel Plan journey. Now trim the list down to only those things you need to deal with today.

DAILY
CHECK-IN

 FOOD

- How did your meals align with The Daniel Plan plate today?

- How would you rate your eating today on a scale of 1 to 10 (10 being best):

1	2	3	4	5	6	7	8	9	10

- Some of the best choices I made today were:
  (e.g., eating a healthy breakfast)

👟 FITNESS

- What type of fitness/movement did you do today?

- Duration:

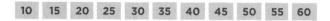

💡 FOCUS

- Gratitude for today:

- Goal for tomorrow:

👥 FRIENDS

- Who encouraged, supported, or joined you on your health journey today?

- Who needs your encouragement, support, or companionship?

DAILY
FOOD TRACKER

- What did you eat? How did it make you feel?

  BREAKFAST:

  SNACK:

  LUNCH:

  SNACK:

  DINNER:

  WATER: HOW MUCH WATER DID YOU DRINK?

- When you ate today, was it because you were hungry? Or were you motivated by boredom, stress, or fatigue?

- What worked?

- Any adjustments or changes for tomorrow?

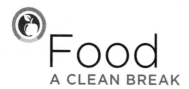

Food
A CLEAN BREAK

Dear friends, let's make a clean break with everything that defiles or distracts us, both within and without. Let's make our entire lives fit and holy temples for the worship of God.
— 2 Corinthians 7:1 MSG

DAILY
REFLECTION

Becoming healthy involves gradual progress, but you can make an immediate change by starting with your kitchen. You may be surprised to discover how many unhealthy ingredients and health food impostors are lurking in your pantry.

Very few of us would open the sugar canister and scoop a spoonful as a snack. But many of us do the equivalent of that when we grab snacks like a granola bar without ever investigating the label. For example, refined flour, high fructose corn syrup, and other menaces are often "hidden in plain sight" in our food.

It's time for a clean break. Clear out the bad to make way for the healthy abundance of foods that are a part of The Daniel Plan.

Today, take inventory of the food you have on hand in your

pantry and fridge. Make a goal to remove all foods with ingredients that you don't recognize as real food.

Why do you think it's necessary to clean out your pantry?

 FAITH

- Besides taste, what is it about unhealthy foods that appeals to you? Have you ever talked to God about your food habits and cravings? How do you need to change your thinking so that your health is more important than convenience?

DAILY
CHECK-IN

 FOOD

- How did your meals align with The Daniel Plan plate today?

- How would you rate your eating today on a scale of 1 to 10 (10 being best):

| 1 | 2 | 3 | 4 | 5 | 6 | 7 | 8 | 9 | 10 |

- Some of the best choices I made today were:
  (e.g., eating a healthy breakfast)

🥾 FITNESS

- What type of fitness/movement did you do today?

- Duration:

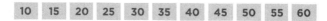

💡 FOCUS

- Gratitude for today:

- Goal for tomorrow:

👥 FRIENDS

- Who encouraged, supported, or joined you on your health journey today?

- Who needs your encouragement, support, or companionship?

DAILY
FOOD TRACKER

- What did you eat? How did it make you feel?

    BREAKFAST:

    SNACK:

    LUNCH:

    SNACK:

    DINNER:

    WATER: HOW MUCH WATER DID YOU DRINK?

- When you ate today, was it because you were hungry?
  Or were you motivated by boredom, stress, or fatigue?

- What worked?

- Any adjustments or changes for tomorrow?

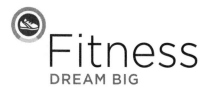

Fitness
DREAM BIG

With God's power working in us, God can do much, much more than anything we can ask or imagine.
— *Ephesians 3:20 NCV*

DAILY
REFLECTION

If you can reach your dreams without God, then they're just not big enough. God wants to give you dreams that are so huge and audacious that they can only come true through his mighty power.

God will use your dreams to push you past your comfort zone and believe you can achieve your fitness goals. He will use your fitness dreams to keep you from simply settling for so-so results. It may feel risky to dream big, but ultimately your dreams are up to God.

What are the obstacles that might keep you from accomplishing your goals

> "Every great dream begins with a dreamer. Always remember, you have within you the strength, the patience, and the passion to reach for the stars to change the world."
> —Harriet Tubman

and dreams? What are your solutions to overcoming those obstacles?

FAITH

- What is your Big Fitness Dream (e.g., run a 10K or climb a mountain)? If you don't have a Big Fitness Dream, ask God to give you one — and then expect him to answer.

DAILY
CHECK-IN

FOOD

- How did your meals align with The Daniel Plan plate today?

- How would you rate your eating today on a scale of 1 to 10 (10 being best):

| 1 | 2 | 3 | 4 | 5 | 6 | 7 | 8 | 9 | 10 |

- Some of the best choices I made today were:
  (e.g., eating a healthy breakfast)

🏃 FITNESS

- What type of fitness/movement did you do today?

- Duration:

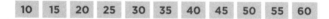

💡 FOCUS

- Gratitude for today:

- Goal for tomorrow:

👥 FRIENDS

- Who encouraged, supported, or joined you on your health journey today?

- Who needs your encouragement, support, or companionship?

DAILY
FOOD TRACKER

- What did you eat? How did it make you feel?

   BREAKFAST:

   SNACK:

   LUNCH:

   SNACK:

   DINNER:

   WATER: HOW MUCH WATER DID YOU DRINK?

- When you ate today, was it because you were hungry?
  Or were you motivated by boredom, stress, or fatigue?

- What worked?

- Any adjustments or changes for tomorrow?

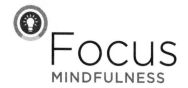

Focus
MINDFULNESS

Set your minds on things above, not on earthly things.
— *Colossians 3:2*

DAILY
REFLECTION

Many of us believe we can multi-task without limits. However our brain isn't a computer; it can't run different programs simultaneously. When we think we are "multi-tasking," we are actually switching rapidly between tasks. Our attention is divided. That's why people sometimes crash their cars when they try to text and drive.

It's also often why people crash in their journey to get healthy. Getting healthy the right way requires that you approach each task with mindfulness of God's priorities. You must focus on what's most important and not allow yourself to get distracted by the trivial.

As you make the commitment to set your mind on the things God has for you, you will be able to lay aside what doesn't matter and focus on his plan for your body.

🏋 FAITH

- Make a list of all the things you have to do in a typical day or week. Pray over each task, obligation, and chore, asking for God's priorities to guide you.

- Are you struggling to give undivided attention to the people and things in your life to which God has called you? What are the things that distract you from what's important?

- Is God asking you to give up anything?

DAILY
CHECK-IN

🍎 FOOD

- How did your meals align with The Daniel Plan plate today?

- How would you rate your eating today on a scale of 1 to 10 (10 being best):

| 1 | 2 | 3 | 4 | 5 | 6 | 7 | 8 | 9 | 10 |

- Some of the best choices I made today were:
  (e.g., eating a healthy breakfast)

🏃 FITNESS

- What type of fitness/movement did you do today?

- Duration:

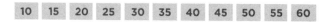

💡 FOCUS

- Gratitude for today:

- Goal for tomorrow:

👥 FRIENDS

- Who encouraged, supported, or joined you on your health journey today?

- Who needs your encouragement, support, or companionship?

DAILY
FOOD TRACKER

- What did you eat? How did it make you feel?

  BREAKFAST:

  SNACK:

  LUNCH:

  SNACK:

  DINNER:

  WATER: HOW MUCH WATER DID YOU DRINK?

- When you ate today, was it because you were hungry?
  Or were you motivated by boredom, stress, or fatigue?

- What worked?

- Any adjustments or changes for tomorrow?

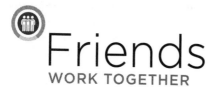

Friends
WORK TOGETHER

And let us consider how we may spur one another on toward love and good deeds.

— *Hebrews 10:24*

DAILY
REFLECTION

Real friends bring out the best in each other. They encourage and motivate one another to reach their goals. Friends who will cheer you on to success are a critical part of The Daniel Plan.

There is an old Zambian proverb that says, "When you run alone, you run fast. But when you run together, you run far." The Daniel Plan — and the lifetime of healthy habits ahead of you — is a journey of distance, not a fifty-yard dash.

When you want to give up, if you have friends running with you, you can find the strength to go the distance. Friends will help you achieve your God-given health goals.

Why do you think it's important to want your friends' success as much as your own?

🌀 FAITH

- We all have different strengths when it comes to encouraging others. What are some ways you can encourage your friends on The Daniel Plan?

- Write Romans 12:5 on a note card, and put it in a place you will look at frequently as an encouragement when you are struggling with your Daniel Plan commitments. Whose phone number can you add to the note card to easily reach out for help?

DAILY
CHECK-IN

🌀 FOOD

- How did your meals align with The Daniel Plan plate today?

- How would you rate your eating today on a scale of 1 to 10 (10 being best):

1   2   3   4   5   6   7   8   9   10

- Some of the best choices I made today were:
  (*e.g., eating a healthy breakfast*)

👟 FITNESS

- What type of fitness/movement did you do today?

- Duration:

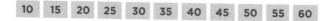

| 10 | 15 | 20 | 25 | 30 | 35 | 40 | 45 | 50 | 55 | 60 |

💡 FOCUS

- Gratitude for today:

- Goal for tomorrow:

👥 FRIENDS

- Who encouraged, supported, or joined you on your
  health journey today?

- Who needs your encouragement, support, or
  companionship?

DAILY
FOOD TRACKER

- What did you eat? How did it make you feel?

  BREAKFAST:

  SNACK:

  LUNCH:

  SNACK:

  DINNER:

  WATER: HOW MUCH WATER DID YOU DRINK?

- When you ate today, was it because you were hungry? Or were you motivated by boredom, stress, or fatigue?

- What worked?

- Any adjustments or changes for tomorrow?

10-Day Check-In

	DAY 10
Height	
Weight	
BMI*	
Blood Pressure	
Waist	
Hips	
Activity Level**	

*Refer to page 199 to calculate your BMI.
**Sedentary (I rarely or never do any physical activities)
Light (I do some light or moderate physical activities every week)
Regular (I do moderate physical activities every week, 20–30 minutes a day for 3–4 days a week)
Active to vigorous (I do moderate to vigorous physical activities every week, 30–60 minutes a day for 5 or more days a week)

PERSONAL
ASSESSMENT

FAITH   FOOD   FITNESS   FOCUS   FRIENDS

- What Essentials have you been focusing on, and why?

- What progress have you made? *Celebrate your wins!*

- Is something still standing in your way? If so, what will you do differently to overcome it?

- What is something new you have learned about yourself?

- Based on what you have learned, what will you change next week?

- Already achieved your goals? *Congratulations!* It's time to set some new goals.

- Circle one to two *new* Essentials to focus on for the next ten days.

  FAITH   FOOD   FITNESS   FOCUS   FRIENDS

- Now set your SMART Goals, and share them with a friend!

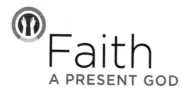

Faith
A PRESENT GOD

*"Do not be afraid or discouraged, for the L*ORD
will personally go ahead of you. He will be with you;
he will neither fail you nor abandon you."

— Deuteronomy 31:8 NLT

DAILY
REFLECTION

God promises to be with you every step of the way as you work to become Daniel Strong. He won't let you down, and he won't abandon you. When you struggle on your journey, remember that God is right there with you. This isn't just a feel-good, figurative statement — God is present, now and forever.

If you are discouraged, the answer isn't for you to try harder not to be discouraged. The answer is to trust that God is true to his Word. For example, when you start to worry, say, "I choose not to worry in this moment because I trust God is clearing the path before me." You increase your faith by taking a step — no matter how small — to trust in God's promises.

FAITH

- How will believing God is with you every single step change your mind and change your health?

- When have you seen God help you in your faith or your trust or your journey toward better health? Write down your observations, and continue to add to them as you see God at work in your life.

DAILY
CHECK-IN

FOOD

- How did your meals align with The Daniel Plan plate today?

- How would you rate your eating today on a scale of 1 to 10 (10 being best):

- Some of the best choices I made today were:
  (e.g., eating a healthy breakfast)

👟 FITNESS

- What type of fitness/movement did you do today?

- Duration:

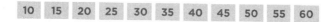

| 10 | 15 | 20 | 25 | 30 | 35 | 40 | 45 | 50 | 55 | 60 |

💡 FOCUS

- Gratitude for today:

- Goal for tomorrow:

👥 FRIENDS

- Who encouraged, supported, or joined you on your health journey today?

- Who needs your encouragement, support, or companionship?

DAILY
FOOD TRACKER

- What did you eat? How did it make you feel?

  BREAKFAST:

  SNACK:

  LUNCH:

  SNACK:

  DINNER:

  WATER: HOW MUCH WATER DID YOU DRINK?

- When you ate today, was it because you were hungry?
  Or were you motivated by boredom, stress, or fatigue?

- What worked?

- Any adjustments or changes for tomorrow?

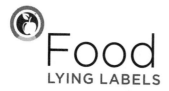

Food
LYING LABELS

*Be very careful, then, how you live —
not as unwise but as wise.*
— Ephesians 5:15

DAILY
REFLECTION

One of the things you are learning in your efforts to become healthier is that real change requires you to face the truth and the lies.

Changing eating habits begins with developing discernment. If a food is labeled "healthy" but has 20 ingredients, 19 of which you can't pronounce, that label is lying. Educate yourself about what is truly healthful food, such as fresh vegetables, lean meat, nuts, and fruit.

While it may seem confusing at first — shouldn't you be able to trust any food that is labeled "healthy," "all natural," "diet," or "fat-free"? — it is really quite simple to eat healthy. Once you learn to recognize lying labels, you will be empowered to make the best choices for your body.

God wants you to "use your head — and heart! — to discern what is right, to test what is authentically right" (John 7:24 MSG).

What are some of the surprising things you've learned so far about lying labels?

🏋 FAITH

- What changes do you and your family need to make so you can cultivate the habit of reading labels? How can you seek God's wisdom when it comes to your food choices?

- Think about and talk about this statement with your small group or friends: "I've come to look at this process as embracing healthy choices rather than denying myself" (Lysa TerKeurst).

DAILY
CHECK-IN

🌀 FOOD

- How did your meals align with The Daniel Plan plate today?

- How would you rate your eating today on a scale of 1 to 10 (10 being best):

| 1 | 2 | 3 | 4 | 5 | 6 | 7 | 8 | 9 | 10 |

- Some of the best choices I made today were:
  (*e.g., eating a healthy breakfast*)

🅢 FITNESS

- What type of fitness/movement did you do today?

- Duration:

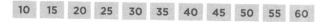

💡 FOCUS

- Gratitude for today:

- Goal for tomorrow:

👪 FRIENDS

- Who encouraged, supported, or joined you on your
  health journey today?

- Who needs your encouragement, support, or
  companionship?

DAILY
FOOD TRACKER

- What did you eat? How did it make you feel?

  BREAKFAST:

  SNACK:

  LUNCH:

  SNACK:

  DINNER:

  WATER: HOW MUCH WATER DID YOU DRINK?

- When you ate today, was it because you were hungry? Or were you motivated by boredom, stress, or fatigue?

- What worked?

- Any adjustments or changes for tomorrow?

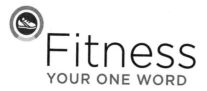

Fitness
YOUR ONE WORD

My son, pay attention to what I say; turn your ear to my words. Do not let them out of your sight, keep them within your heart; for they are life to those who find them and health to one's whole body.

— *Proverbs 4:20 – 22*

DAILY
REFLECTION

In their book *One Word That Will Change Your Life*, authors Dan Britton, Jimmy Page, and Jon Gordon write about how spending an entire year focused on one word, such as *serving, grace, purpose,* or *surrender,* can change your life.*

They say, "Just as a light focused becomes a laser that can cut through steel, a life focused with One Word becomes a force that can cut through the status quo."

Think about your fitness goals, and then ask God what one word should be your focus for just next week. With that word, focus yourself on becoming Daniel Strong.

Today, go for a walk and look for a small, smooth, flat stone.

---

*Dan Britton, Jimmy Page, and Jon Gordon, *One Word That Will Change Your Life* (Hoboken, NJ: Wiley and Sons, 2013).

Write your "one word" on the stone with a permanent marker. Carry it with you or put it someplace where you will see it regularly, and watch how God will use it to make you Daniel Strong.

What word did you choose for your fitness? What does it mean?

🎭 FAITH

- How can your one word also help you with your faith?

- What do you hope to gain by focusing on this one word?

DAILY
CHECK-IN

🌀 FOOD

- How did your meals align with The Daniel Plan plate today?

- How would you rate your eating today on a scale of 1 to 10 (10 being best):

1   2   3   4   5   6   7   8   9   10

- Some of the best choices I made today were:
  (e.g., eating a healthy breakfast)

🏃 FITNESS

- What type of fitness/movement did you do today?

- Duration:

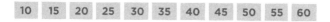

💡 FOCUS

- Gratitude for today:

- Goal for tomorrow:

👥 FRIENDS

- Who encouraged, supported, or joined you on your health journey today?

- Who needs your encouragement, support, or companionship?

DAILY
FOOD TRACKER

- What did you eat? How did it make you feel?

    BREAKFAST:

    SNACK:

    LUNCH:

    SNACK:

    DINNER:

    WATER: HOW MUCH WATER DID YOU DRINK?

- When you ate today, was it because you were hungry? Or were you motivated by boredom, stress, or fatigue?

- What worked?

- Any adjustments or changes for tomorrow?

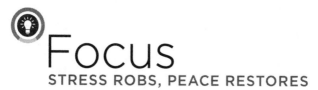

Focus
STRESS ROBS, PEACE RESTORES

You will keep in perfect peace all who trust in you,
all whose thoughts are fixed on you!
— Isaiah 26:3 NLT

DAILY
REFLECTION

As you work to renew your mind, stress will undoubtedly try to pull you away from your goals. The problems of everyday life often tempt us to make unhealthy choices out of convenience or as a temporary fix for handling stress.

But the truth is, problems will follow you the rest of your life. If you're waiting to deal with stress until you make it to a new stage in your life, you will be waiting a long time!

Stress robs us of God's peace and clarity. We get stressed out when we focus on our own limited resources instead of focusing on the unlimited resources through our heavenly Father.

When we choose to focus on God, he strengthens us with his perfect peace. He helps us to stay balanced, focused, and strong. Focus on the fact that God is big enough to get you through any challenges you face.

What causes you the greatest stress?

🎭 FAITH

- Now fix your thoughts on God for five to ten minutes. How does this help? What keeps you from focusing on God?

- What are some practical ways you can turn your mind toward Christ daily to find his peace?

DAILY
CHECK-IN

🍃 FOOD

- How did your meals align with The Daniel Plan plate today?

- How would you rate your eating today on a scale of 1 to 10 (10 being best):

1   2   3   4   5   6   7   8   9   10

- Some of the best choices I made today were:
  (e.g., eating a healthy breakfast)

🥾 FITNESS

- What type of fitness/movement did you do today?

- Duration:

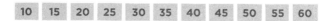

💡 FOCUS

- Gratitude for today:

- Goal for tomorrow:

👥 FRIENDS

- Who encouraged, supported, or joined you on your health journey today?

- Who needs your encouragement, support, or companionship?

DAILY
FOOD TRACKER

- What did you eat? How did it make you feel?

  BREAKFAST:

  SNACK:

  LUNCH:

  SNACK:

  DINNER:

  WATER: HOW MUCH WATER DID YOU DRINK?

- When you ate today, was it because you were hungry? Or were you motivated by boredom, stress, or fatigue?

- What worked?

- Any adjustments or changes for tomorrow?

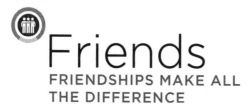

Friends
FRIENDSHIPS MAKE ALL THE DIFFERENCE

There is no fear in love.
But perfect love drives out fear…
— 1 John 4:18

DAILY
REFLECTION

Many people are afraid to get close to others, even their friends, because they are concerned that if others see who they really are, they will be rejected.

God's answer to fear is love. God enables us to love the fear out of one another.

We drive fear from our community by loving one another so supportively that each person feels safe inside the group. This safety allows us to bring our humanity into the group, including all our joy and pain, our ups and downs, our victories and defeats. That is what deep and committed friendships offer — and everyone needs them.

When was a time your friends made you stronger? How have you been able to offer strength and commitment to some of your friends?

FAITH

- Why are you sometimes afraid to let others see the real you? Ask God to help you work through those fears and lower any walls so you can let your friends see the real you.

DAILY
CHECK-IN

FOOD

- How did your meals align with The Daniel Plan plate today?

- How would you rate your eating today on a scale of 1 to 10 (10 being best):

| 1 | 2 | 3 | 4 | 5 | 6 | 7 | 8 | 9 | 10 |

- Some of the best choices I made today were:
  (e.g., eating a healthy breakfast)

🥿 FITNESS

- What type of fitness/movement did you do today?

- Duration:

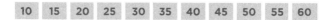

💡 FOCUS

- Gratitude for today:

- Goal for tomorrow:

👥 FRIENDS

- Who encouraged, supported, or joined you on your health journey today?

- Who needs your encouragement, support, or companionship?

DAILY
FOOD TRACKER

- What did you eat? How did it make you feel?

   BREAKFAST:

   SNACK:

   LUNCH:

   SNACK:

   DINNER:

   WATER: HOW MUCH WATER DID YOU DRINK?

- When you ate today, was it because you were hungry? Or were you motivated by boredom, stress, or fatigue?

- What worked?

- Any adjustments or changes for tomorrow?

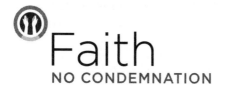

Faith
NO CONDEMNATION

So now there is no condemnation for those
who belong to Christ Jesus.
                    — Romans 8:1 NLT

DAILY
REFLECTION

Did you know God knows that you will fail unless you are intimately connected to him? He is not surprised when you stumble on your way.

God doesn't expect us to be perfect. In fact, he uses our failures to show us that we need him and to drive us into his arms of grace.

There is no condemnation for those who belong to Christ Jesus! This means that no matter how bad you blow it in life or on The Daniel Plan, God will never condemn you. He not only wants you to succeed, but is also actively working with every setback to help you succeed.

FAITH

- What reasons make you feel as if you need to be perfect with The Daniel Plan? Does God expect you to be perfect?

- Write down some of the mistakes or setbacks you have had so far on your journey toward better health. Use just one or two words to identify them. Then write "NO CONDEMNATION" next to each entry on the list. Pray through the list, and thank God that you are forgiven and that he goes before you.

DAILY
CHECK-IN

 FOOD

- How did your meals align with The Daniel Plan plate today?

- How would you rate your eating today on a scale of 1 to 10 (10 being best):

  1   2   3   4   5   6   7   8   9   10

- Some of the best choices I made today were:
  (e.g., eating a healthy breakfast)

👟 FITNESS

- What type of fitness/movement did you do today?

- Duration:

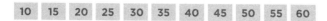

💡 FOCUS

- Gratitude for today:

- Goal for tomorrow:

👥 FRIENDS

- Who encouraged, supported, or joined you on your health journey today?

- Who needs your encouragement, support, or companionship?

DAILY
FOOD TRACKER

- What did you eat? How did it make you feel?

  BREAKFAST:

  SNACK:

  LUNCH:

  SNACK:

  DINNER:

  WATER: HOW MUCH WATER DID YOU DRINK?

- When you ate today, was it because you were hungry? Or were you motivated by boredom, stress, or fatigue?

- What worked?

- Any adjustments or changes for tomorrow?

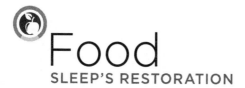

Food
SLEEP'S RESTORATION

God gives rest to his loved ones.
— *Psalm 127:2 NLT*

DAILY
REFLECTION

When you sleep, your heavenly Father watches over you in love. Sleep is God's gift. To accept that gift is an act of trust. He restores your body and energy through sleep.

One of the hidden triggers to overeating is lack of rest. When we are overtired, we often try to boost our energy with caffeine, sugar, or carbs, which ultimately leaves us more tired than before.

Restful sleep gives us the energy to exercise. It sharpens our focus and helps us to make good choices about food.

Jesus relaxed, and he offered his followers both physical and spiritual rest. If he didn't sacrifice rest but offered it as a gift, shouldn't we accept that gift? Turn to him for rest.

How might a good night's sleep help you meet your Daniel Plan goals?

FAITH

- Matthew 11:28 – 29 says, "Come to me, all you who are weary and burdened, and I will give you rest. Take my yoke upon you and learn from me, for I am gentle and humble in heart, and you will find rest for your souls." What longings stir in you when you read Jesus' invitation to rest?

DAILY
CHECK-IN

FOOD

- How did your meals align with The Daniel Plan plate today?

- How would you rate your eating today on a scale of 1 to 10 (10 being best):

  | 1 | 2 | 3 | 4 | 5 | 6 | 7 | 8 | 9 | 10 |

- Some of the best choices I made today were:
  (e.g., eating a healthy breakfast)

FITNESS

- What type of fitness/movement did you do today?

- Duration:

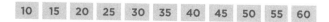

FOCUS

- Gratitude for today:

- Goal for tomorrow:

FRIENDS

- Who encouraged, supported, or joined you on your
  health journey today?

- Who needs your encouragement, support, or
  companionship?

DAILY
FOOD TRACKER

- What did you eat? How did it make you feel?

  BREAKFAST:

  SNACK:

  LUNCH:

  SNACK:

  DINNER:

  WATER: HOW MUCH WATER DID YOU DRINK?

- When you ate today, was it because you were hungry?
  Or were you motivated by boredom, stress, or fatigue?

- What worked?

- Any adjustments or changes for tomorrow?

Fitness
YOUR AMAZING
AND WONDERFUL BODY

*You made my whole being; you formed me in my
mother's body. I praise you because you made me
in an amazing and wonderful way. What you have
done is wonderful. I know this very well.*
— Psalm 139:13–14 NCV

DAILY
REFLECTION

God made you in an amazing and wonderful way! He sees you
as a work of art. He does not look at you critically, but with deep
love. Our bodies are his workmanship.

Knowing that truth, what is the right attitude toward your
body? Don't reject it, and don't neglect it.

Keeping your body in shape is a spiritual discipline. God
created your body. Jesus died for it. The Holy Spirit lives in it.
Your body is connected to Christ, and it's going to be resur-
rected one day. On that day God will hold you accountable for
how you managed your body. But he doesn't leave you alone to
do that. He is with you every step of your journey.

FAITH

- God gave you the body that you will need to complete your mission here on earth. How does that change the way you look at your body?

- Write a short description of yourself here. What are the strengths God has given you? What can you do with those strengths for God's glory?

DAILY
CHECK-IN

FOOD

- How did your meals align with The Daniel Plan plate today?

- How would you rate your eating today on a scale of 1 to 10 (10 being best):

  1   2   3   4   5   6   7   8   9   10

- Some of the best choices I made today were:
  (e.g., eating a healthy breakfast)

🥾 FITNESS

- What type of fitness/movement did you do today?

- Duration:

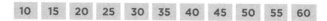

💡 FOCUS

- Gratitude for today:

- Goal for tomorrow:

👥 FRIENDS

- Who encouraged, supported, or joined you on your
  health journey today?

- Who needs your encouragement, support, or
  companionship?

DAILY
FOOD TRACKER

- What did you eat? How did it make you feel?

   BREAKFAST:

   SNACK:

   LUNCH:

   SNACK:

   DINNER:

   WATER: HOW MUCH WATER DID YOU DRINK?

- When you ate today, was it because you were hungry? Or were you motivated by boredom, stress, or fatigue?

- What worked?

- Any adjustments or changes for tomorrow?

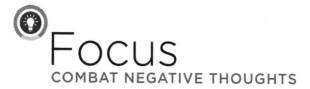

Focus
COMBAT NEGATIVE THOUGHTS

Be careful what you think, because your thoughts run your life.
— *Proverbs 4:23 NCV*

DAILY
REFLECTION

Changing your health habits is like driving a speedboat on a lake with your automatic pilot set to go east. If you want to reverse course, you could try to physically force the wheel in the opposite direction, but you would likely get tired and let go, and the boat would drift back.

There is a better option: Change your autopilot. The same is true with your health habits. To make a lasting change, you must change how you think. Behind everything you do — even your unhealthy habits — is a thought that keeps you from getting healthy. Instead, the Bible says you should "have the same mindset as Christ Jesus" (Philippians 2:5).

God wants you to learn to think like Jesus. How do you do that? You meditate on God's Word and you ask, "Lord, how would Jesus think about this?" The more you fill your mind with the Word of God, the sooner you reset your autopilot in the direction of truth.

FAITH

- What are some of the beliefs that have derailed your attempts to get healthy in the past?

- What are some truths from God's Word that can change the autopilot that keeps you from getting healthy?

- What do you need to change about the way you do your quiet time or structure your schedule so that you can fill your mind with the Word of God?

DAILY
CHECK-IN

FOOD

- How did your meals align with The Daniel Plan plate today?

- How would you rate your eating today on a scale of 1 to 10 (10 being best):

| 1 | 2 | 3 | 4 | 5 | 6 | 7 | 8 | 9 | 10 |

- Some of the best choices I made today were:
  (e.g., eating a healthy breakfast)

👟 FITNESS

- What type of fitness/movement did you do today?

- Duration:

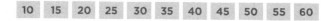

💡 FOCUS

- Gratitude for today:

- Goal for tomorrow:

👥 FRIENDS

- Who encouraged, supported, or joined you on your health journey today?

- Who needs your encouragement, support, or companionship?

DAILY
FOOD TRACKER

- What did you eat? How did it make you feel?

   BREAKFAST:

   SNACK:

   LUNCH:

   SNACK:

   DINNER:

   WATER: HOW MUCH WATER DID YOU DRINK?

- When you ate today, was it because you were hungry?
  Or were you motivated by boredom, stress, or fatigue?

- What worked?

- Any adjustments or changes for tomorrow?

Friends
GOOD FRIENDS ARE GOOD LISTENERS

My dear brothers and sisters, always be willing to listen and slow to speak.

— James 1:19 NCV

DAILY
REFLECTION

An important step toward deepening friendships is to learn to be quick to listen and slow to speak.

When you take time to listen to others, it tells them how important they are to you. By letting them get their story out and not jumping in to try to fix them, you provide a safe place for them to express their frustrations and fears.

Consider this: God patiently listens to you, even though he already knows what you are going to say. He doesn't cut you off or rush you through your thoughts. He's not afraid of your anger, and his response is thoughtful and in your best interest. If the God of the universe does this for you, should you do any less for your friends?

How can you become a safe listener within your group? What characteristics will make you a good listener?

FAITH

- Part of being a good listener is asking questions. The Bible says, "Knowing what is right is like deep water in the heart; a wise person draws from the well within" (Proverbs 20:5 MSG). What kind of questions can you ask that will draw a person out?

DAILY
CHECK-IN

FOOD

- How did your meals align with The Daniel Plan plate today?

- How would you rate your eating today on a scale of 1 to 10 (10 being best):

| 1 | 2 | 3 | 4 | 5 | 6 | 7 | 8 | 9 | 10 |

- Some of the best choices I made today were:
  (e.g., eating a healthy breakfast)

🥾 FITNESS

- What type of fitness/movement did you do today?

- Duration:

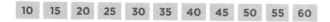

  10 15 20 25 30 35 40 45 50 55 60

💡 FOCUS

- Gratitude for today:

- Goal for tomorrow:

👪 FRIENDS

- Who encouraged, supported, or joined you on your
  health journey today?

- Who needs your encouragement, support, or
  companionship?

DAILY
FOOD TRACKER

- What did you eat? How did it make you feel?

  BREAKFAST:

  SNACK:

  LUNCH:

  SNACK:

  DINNER:

  WATER: HOW MUCH WATER DID YOU DRINK?

- When you ate today, was it because you were hungry?
  Or were you motivated by boredom, stress, or fatigue?

- What worked?

- Any adjustments or changes for tomorrow?

10-Day Check-In

	DAY 20
Height	
Weight	
BMI*	
Blood Pressure	
Waist	
Hips	
Activity Level**	

*Refer to page 199 to calculate your BMI.

Sedentary (I rarely or never do any physical activities)

Light (I do some light or moderate physical activities every week)

Regular (I do moderate physical activities every week, 20–30 minutes a day for 3–4 days a week)

Active to vigorous (I do moderate to vigorous physical activities every week, 30–60 minutes a day for 5 or more days a week)

PERSONAL
ASSESSMENT

FAITH

FOOD

FITNESS

FOCUS

FRIENDS

- What Essentials have you been focusing on, and why?

- What progress have you made? *Celebrate your wins!*

- Is something still standing in your way? If so, what will you do differently to overcome it?

- What is something new you have learned about yourself?

- Based on what you have learned, what will you change next week?

- Already achieved your goals? *Congratulations!* It's time to set some new goals.

- Circle one to two *new* Essentials to focus on for the next ten days.

  FAITH   FOOD   FITNESS   FOCUS   FRIENDS

- Now set your SMART Goals, and share them with a friend!

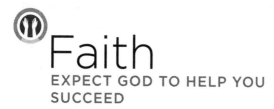

Faith

EXPECT GOD TO HELP YOU SUCCEED

"According to your faith let it be done to you."
— *Matthew 9:29*

DAILY
REFLECTION

How are you expecting God to help you on your journey toward better health? Faith is expecting God to fulfill his promises and help you do what he has called you to do. It is the difference between thinking, *God* might *help me get healthier* and *God* will *help me get healthier.*

Faith means you are certain that God is there, helping you every step along the way. It means you are certain that God not only wants you to succeed, but that he's also actively working for your success.

Talk to God about your journey, including your hopes, your fears, your concerns, and your expectations. He will respond according to your faith.

FAITH

- When you pray, do you "sort of" hope God will answer your prayer, or do you expect him to answer?

- How do you expect him to help you on your journey with The Daniel Plan?

- Ask God to give you a vision of what your life will be like as you become healthier. Then write down what he reveals to you in his time.

DAILY
CHECK-IN

FOOD

- How did your meals align with The Daniel Plan plate today?

- How would you rate your eating today on a scale of 1 to 10 (10 being best):

| 1 | 2 | 3 | 4 | 5 | 6 | 7 | 8 | 9 | 10 |

- Some of the best choices I made today were:
  (e.g., eating a healthy breakfast)

🏃 FITNESS

- What type of fitness/movement did you do today?

- Duration:

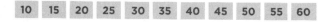

💡 FOCUS

- Gratitude for today:

- Goal for tomorrow:

👥 FRIENDS

- Who encouraged, supported, or joined you on your health journey today?

- Who needs your encouragement, support, or companionship?

DAILY
FOOD TRACKER

- What did you eat? How did it make you feel?

    BREAKFAST:

    SNACK:

    LUNCH:

    SNACK:

    DINNER:

    WATER: HOW MUCH WATER DID YOU DRINK?

- When you ate today, was it because you were hungry? Or were you motivated by boredom, stress, or fatigue?

- What worked?

- Any adjustments or changes for tomorrow?

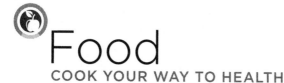

Food

COOK YOUR WAY TO HEALTH

When they landed, they saw a fire of burning coals there with fish on it, and some bread. Jesus said to them, "Bring some of the fish you have just caught.... Come and have breakfast...." Jesus came, took the bread and gave it to them, and did the same with the fish.
— *John 21:9 – 10, 12 – 13*

DAILY
REFLECTION

How would you feel if Jesus cooked you a meal? The Bible gives a snapshot of Jesus cooking a simple meal on the beach using fresh food. Jesus took the time to cook — for his friends.

You can ask Jesus to join you as you prepare a meal, talking to him and praising him for supporting you on the road to better health.

If you want to change the way that you eat, the logical place to begin is to change the way you cook. Cooking is not nearly as complicated as

> "Cooking is at once child's play and adult joy. And cooking done with care is an act of love."
> —Craig Claiborne, former *New York Times* Food Editor

people sometimes believe it to be. And when you combine it with deepening your relationship with Jesus and making it an act of worship, it can become extraordinary.

How does cooking food impact your experience of eating it?

FAITH

- If you were cooking with Jesus, what's the first meal you would make? Find a simple meal that you think would be appropriate and fun, and give it a try.

DAILY
CHECK-IN

FOOD

- How did your meals align with The Daniel Plan plate today?

- How would you rate your eating today on a scale of 1 to 10 (10 being best):

- Some of the best choices I made today were:
  (e.g., eating a healthy breakfast)

FITNESS

- What type of fitness/movement did you do today?

- Duration:

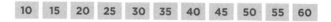

10   15   20   25   30   35   40   45   50   55   60

FOCUS

- Gratitude for today:

- Goal for tomorrow:

FRIENDS

- Who encouraged, supported, or joined you on your
  health journey today?

- Who needs your encouragement, support, or
  companionship?

DAILY
FOOD TRACKER

- What did you eat? How did it make you feel?

  BREAKFAST:

  SNACK:

  LUNCH:

  SNACK:

  DINNER:

  WATER: HOW MUCH WATER DID YOU DRINK?

- When you ate today, was it because you were hungry? Or were you motivated by boredom, stress, or fatigue?

- What worked?

- Any adjustments or changes for tomorrow?

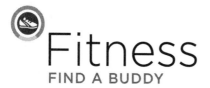

Fitness
FIND A BUDDY

Two are better than one, because they have a good return for their labor: If either of them falls down, one can help the other up. But pity anyone who falls and has no one to help them up.
— *Ecclesiastes 4:9–10*

DAILY
REFLECTION

Working out with a friend helps you be more consistent in your exercise, stick with each session longer, and even burn more calories! A workout buddy will encourage you, keep you accountable, and push you to reach your goals. If you work out with someone a bit stronger and fitter than you, just trying to keep up will improve your fitness level.

When you exercise with a friend, you help each other prepare to serve God with more stamina and energy. Having an exercise buddy also provides you another wonderful opportunity: the chance to help someone else. You will improve your fitness and experience the joy of friendship, both of which will help you to become Daniel Strong.

How would a fitness buddy help you stay motivated and reach your goals?

FAITH

- Ask God who could be a fitness partner for you. Who could you join on his or her fitness journey?

DAILY
CHECK-IN

FOOD

- How did your meals align with The Daniel Plan plate today?

- How would you rate your eating today on a scale of 1 to 10 (10 being best):

1 2 3 4 5 6 7 8 9 10

- Some of the best choices I made today were:
  (*e.g., eating a healthy breakfast*)

FITNESS

- What type of fitness/movement did you do today?

- Duration:

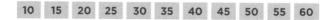

FOCUS

- Gratitude for today:

- Goal for tomorrow:

FRIENDS

- Who encouraged, supported, or joined you on your
  health journey today?

- Who needs your encouragement, support, or
  companionship?

DAILY
FOOD TRACKER

- What did you eat? How did it make you feel?

    BREAKFAST:

    SNACK:

    LUNCH:

    SNACK:

    DINNER:

    WATER: HOW MUCH WATER DID YOU DRINK?

- When you ate today, was it because you were hungry? Or were you motivated by boredom, stress, or fatigue?

- What worked?

- Any adjustments or changes for tomorrow?

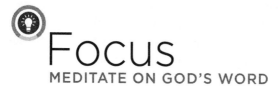

Focus
MEDITATE ON GOD'S WORD

I honor and love your commands.
I meditate on your decrees.
        — Psalm 119:48 NLT

DAILY
REFLECTION

The temptation to abandon the healthy habits you are learning through The Daniel Plan can be quite strong at times. Your only chance to overcome those temptations is to follow the model of Jesus. When he was tempted as related in Matthew 4:1 – 11, Jesus responded with Scripture.

Jesus meditated on and memorized God's Word. Biblical meditation is not about emptying your mind, but filling it with truth. It simply means to read a passage of Scripture, think about it, and repeat it to yourself. It's the first and most important step to remembering and memorizing Bible verses.

No habit will help you in the spiritual dynamics of getting healthy more than meditating on and memorizing the Word of God.

🔾 FAITH

- What are some of the temptations you face on your Daniel Plan journey? Do you struggle with your eating habits when you're stressed? Does your exercise routine suffer when you become too busy?

- Jesus overcame temptation with Scripture. What are some of God's promises you can memorize to counter-act temptation in your life?

DAILY
CHECK-IN

🔾 FOOD

- How did your meals align with The Daniel Plan plate today?

- How would you rate your eating today on a scale of 1 to 10 (10 being best):

| 1 | 2 | 3 | 4 | 5 | 6 | 7 | 8 | 9 | 10 |

- Some of the best choices I made today were:
  (e.g., eating a healthy breakfast)

👟 FITNESS

- What type of fitness/movement did you do today?

- Duration:

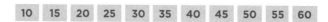

💡 FOCUS

- Gratitude for today:

- Goal for tomorrow:

👥 FRIENDS

- Who encouraged, supported, or joined you on your health journey today?

- Who needs your encouragement, support, or companionship?

DAILY
FOOD TRACKER

- What did you eat? How did it make you feel?

    BREAKFAST:

    SNACK:

    LUNCH:

    SNACK:

    DINNER:

    WATER: HOW MUCH WATER DID YOU DRINK?

- When you ate today, was it because you were hungry? Or were you motivated by boredom, stress, or fatigue?

- What worked?

- Any adjustments or changes for tomorrow?

Friends
SPEAKING THE RIGHT LANGUAGE

If I could speak all the languages of earth and of angels, but didn't love others, I would only be a noisy gong or a clanging cymbal.
— *1 Corinthians 13:1 NLT*

DAILY
REFLECTION

The apostle Paul said that no matter what language we speak, we have to wrap it in love. He added in Romans 13:10, "You can't go wrong when you love others. When you add up everything in the law code, the sum total is *love*" (MSG).

God designed us to reach out to one another and to look out for each other's needs. Loving others well is a sign that we belong to Christ. John 13:35 says, "Your love for one another will prove to the world that you are my disciples" (NLT).

How do you speak the language of love? In his book *The Five Love Languages*, Gary Chapman says each one of us has at least one "language" that makes us feel loved: words of affirmation, receiving gifts, quality time, physical touch, or acts of service.*

*Gary Chapman, *The Five Love Languages* (Chicago: Northfield Press, 1995).

Through which of the five love languages do you feel love? (You may have more than one.)

Write your friends' and family members' names next to the languages that you think speak love to them.

Words of affirmation: _____

Receiving gifts: _____

Quality time: _____

Physical touch: _____

Acts of service: _____

🕊 FAITH

- Put your love into practice. The next time you are with your family, friends, or small group, ask everyone about their love languages. How can you best communicate love to them?

DAILY
CHECK-IN

🍽 FOOD

- How did your meals align with The Daniel Plan plate today?

- How would you rate your eating today on a scale of 1 to 10 (10 being best):

| 1 | 2 | 3 | 4 | 5 | 6 | 7 | 8 | 9 | 10 |

- Some of the best choices I made today were:
  (e.g., eating a healthy breakfast)

👟 FITNESS

- What type of fitness/movement did you do today?

- Duration:

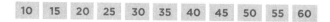

💡 FOCUS

- Gratitude for today:

- Goal for tomorrow:

👥 FRIENDS

- Who encouraged, supported, or joined you on your health journey today?

- Who needs your encouragement, support, or companionship?

DAILY
FOOD TRACKER

- What did you eat? How did it make you feel?

BREAKFAST:

SNACK:

LUNCH:

SNACK:

DINNER:

WATER: HOW MUCH WATER DID YOU DRINK?

- When you ate today, was it because you were hungry?
  Or were you motivated by boredom, stress, or fatigue?

- What worked?

- Any adjustments or changes for tomorrow?

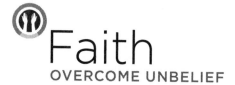

Faith
OVERCOME UNBELIEF

[Asking Jesus to heal his son, the boy's father said,]
"If you can do anything, do it. Have a heart and help
us!" Jesus said, "If? There are no 'ifs' among believers.
Anything can happen." No sooner were the words out
of his mouth than the father cried, "Then I believe.
Help me with my doubts!"

— Mark 9:22 – 24 MSG

DAILY
REFLECTION

Is it possible to have faith and doubts at the same time? Yes! You can have faith that God wants you to do something and still be scared to death. Many of us have thought, "Lord, I have some faith. But I also have some doubts." That's okay, because God lets you begin with the faith you already have. It may be just a little, but you can start there.

Confronting destructive lifelong habits and working toward better physical health will be one of the scariest things some people experience in their lives. Faith is believing that God can do the seemingly impossible in your life, even if you don't understand how.

FAITH

- What are some areas of your life where you trust God is at work?

- What are some areas of your life where you're struggling with doubt, wondering if and how God is really helping you? Bring those concerns to God in prayer.

- How have you already seen God provide for you in your Daniel Plan journey?

DAILY
CHECK-IN

FOOD

- How did your meals align with The Daniel Plan plate today?

- How would you rate your eating today on a scale of 1 to 10 (10 being best):

1 2 3 4 5 6 7 8 9 10

- Some of the best choices I made today were:
  (e.g., eating a healthy breakfast)

👟 FITNESS

- What type of fitness/movement did you do today?

- Duration:

💡 FOCUS

- Gratitude for today:

- Goal for tomorrow:

👥 FRIENDS

- Who encouraged, supported, or joined you on your health journey today?

- Who needs your encouragement, support, or companionship?

DAILY
FOOD TRACKER

- What did you eat? How did it make you feel?

  BREAKFAST:

  SNACK:

  LUNCH:

  SNACK:

  DINNER:

  WATER: HOW MUCH WATER DID YOU DRINK?

- When you ate today, was it because you were hungry? Or were you motivated by boredom, stress, or fatigue?

- What worked?

- Any adjustments or changes for tomorrow?

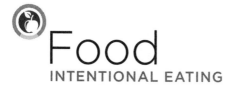

Food
INTENTIONAL EATING

"Please test your servants for ten days: Give us nothing but vegetables to eat and water to drink. Then compare our appearance with that of the young men who eat the royal food, and treat your servants in accordance with what you see." So he agreed to this and tested them for ten days.

At the end of the ten days they looked healthier and better nourished than any of the young men who ate the royal food.

— *Daniel 1:12–15*

DAILY
REFLECTION

Daniel didn't just eat haphazardly, accepting whatever was placed in front of him. He was intentional about what he ate.

When you think clearly about what you eat, God empowers you to continue to make good choices. Clear thinking leads to self-control. By thinking ahead of time, you can prepare so that you won't have a "food emergency." This enables you to eat healthy snacks that you packed ahead of time, and you won't crash in the afternoon because you ate a greasy, fast-food lunch.

Instead, you will be on top of your game, ready to do whatever it is that God calls you to do. Being mindful and conscious, thinking clearly and exercising self-control, you can follow Daniel's example for strength of mind and body.

Write down three things you can do to think clearly and prepare in order to avoid a food emergency.

 FAITH

- What changes do you notice in yourself when you practice mindful and intentional breathing, eating, praying, etc.?

DAILY
CHECK-IN

FOOD

- How did your meals align with The Daniel Plan plate today?

- How would you rate your eating today on a scale of 1 to 10 (10 being best):

| 1 | 2 | 3 | 4 | 5 | 6 | 7 | 8 | 9 | 10 |

- Some of the best choices I made today were:
  (e.g., eating a healthy breakfast)

FITNESS

- What type of fitness/movement did you do today?

- Duration:

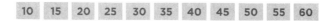

FOCUS

- Gratitude for today:

- Goal for tomorrow:

FRIENDS

- Who encouraged, supported, or joined you on your health journey today?

- Who needs your encouragement, support, or companionship?

DAILY
FOOD TRACKER

- What did you eat? How did it make you feel?

  BREAKFAST:

  SNACK:

  LUNCH:

  SNACK:

  DINNER:

  WATER: HOW MUCH WATER DID YOU DRINK?

- When you ate today, was it because you were hungry? Or were you motivated by boredom, stress, or fatigue?

- What worked?

- Any adjustments or changes for tomorrow?

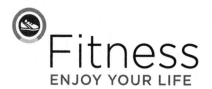

Fitness
ENJOY YOUR LIFE

A cheerful heart is good medicine,
but a crushed spirit dries up the bones.
— *Proverbs 17:22*

DAILY
REFLECTION

God wants you to enjoy life. The apostle Matthew spent three years with Jesus and wrote that he "came, enjoying life" (Matthew 11:19 PH).

After years of being told to stop wiggling and quit fidgeting and work hard, people are very useful but often not very healthy or happy and playful.

It's time to give yourself permission to have fun. Playful behavior is spontaneous and joyful, and in this way it reflects the heart of God.

You can enjoy life because you are secure within God's love. You can have fun, laughing with your friends and family and celebrating the life God has given you.

Take a look at the five statements below relating to play, and identify which statement best describes you.

I like to play because:

1. It's fun!
2. I love competition.
3. I enjoy the personal challenge and accomplishment.
4. I like to learn something new and master it.
5. I just like to be with others.

List a few activities that require you to move your body and that sound like fun.

🎯 FAITH

- Meditate on the truth that Jesus enjoyed life. How does that change your view of him and your understanding of Christianity?

DAILY
CHECK-IN

🍴 FOOD

- How did your meals align with The Daniel Plan plate today?

- How would you rate your eating today on a scale of 1 to 10 (10 being best):

| 1 | 2 | 3 | 4 | 5 | 6 | 7 | 8 | 9 | 10 |

- Some of the best choices I made today were:
  (e.g., eating a healthy breakfast)

🥾 FITNESS

- What type of fitness/movement did you do today?

- Duration:

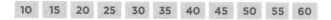

10 15 20 25 30 35 40 45 50 55 60

💡 FOCUS

- Gratitude for today:

- Goal for tomorrow:

👥 FRIENDS

- Who encouraged, supported, or joined you on your health journey today?

- Who needs your encouragement, support, or companionship?

DAILY
FOOD TRACKER

- What did you eat? How did it make you feel?

   BREAKFAST:

   SNACK:

   LUNCH:

   SNACK:

   DINNER:

   WATER: HOW MUCH WATER DID YOU DRINK?

- When you ate today, was it because you were hungry? Or were you motivated by boredom, stress, or fatigue?

- What worked?

- Any adjustments or changes for tomorrow?

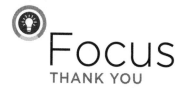

Focus
THANK YOU

Rejoice always, pray continually, give thanks in all circumstances; for this is God's will for you in Christ Jesus.
— *1 Thessalonians 5:16–18*

DAILY
REFLECTION

As God continues to help you grow and get healthier, make a regular practice of telling God "thank you" for what he is doing. You see, one of the healthiest human emotions is gratitude. Gratitude actually increases your immunities. It makes you more resistant to stress and less susceptible to illness. People who are grateful are satisfied with what they have. Cultivating an attitude of gratitude reduces stress in your life and leads to greater spiritual and physical health.

You can't *only* be thankful when your Daniel Plan journey — or life in general — is going well. Gratitude must become a habit, because it will carry you even through difficult times. When you make thankfulness part of your life, you will begin to notice more of what God is doing in and through you.

🦁 FAITH

- Refer back to your Daily Check-Ins to remind yourself of the gratitudes you have recorded for the last 28 days. (Continue recording gratitudes in the Focus section of your Daily Check-In.)

- Ask God to open your eyes to small blessings about each of the trying circumstances in your life. Write a line of gratitude about a few of the challenges you are facing.

DAILY
CHECK-IN

🌱 FOOD

- How did your meals align with The Daniel Plan plate today?

- How would you rate your eating today on a scale of 1 to 10 (10 being best):

1 2 3 4 5 6 7 8 9 10

- Some of the best choices I made today were:
  (e.g., eating a healthy breakfast)

FITNESS

- What type of fitness/movement did you do today?

- Duration:

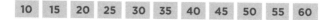

FOCUS

- Gratitude for today:

- Goal for tomorrow:

FRIENDS

- Who encouraged, supported, or joined you on your health journey today?

- Who needs your encouragement, support, or companionship?

DAILY
FOOD TRACKER

- What did you eat? How did it make you feel?

  BREAKFAST:

  SNACK:

  LUNCH:

  SNACK:

  DINNER:

  WATER: HOW MUCH WATER DID YOU DRINK?

- When you ate today, was it because you were hungry?
  Or were you motivated by boredom, stress, or fatigue?

- What worked?

- Any adjustments or changes for tomorrow?

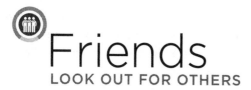

Friends
LOOK OUT FOR OTHERS

Put yourself aside, and help others get ahead.
Don't be obsessed with getting your own advantage.
Forget yourselves long enough to lend a helping hand.
— Philippians 2:4 MSG

DAILY
REFLECTION

It's easy to focus only on yourself as you try to get healthier. Yet, part of becoming like Jesus and improving your health is to get your focus off yourself. The Bible says to put the interests of others above your own. God designed you to look out for others.

Focusing on yourself and your health journey eventually narrows your perspective to only your little world, which can lead you to believe your problems or challenges are worse than anyone else's. That can lead to discouragement. Discouragement can lead to feelings of failure.

But when you focus on others, you see you are not alone, and neither are they. Selflessly work for your friends' success as you would for your own. As you do so, you begin to truly believe that God can help you fulfill your goals because you see so clearly what he is doing in the lives of others.

Make a conscious effort to understand the health goals of your friends, family, or those in your Daniel Plan group. Write those goals down so you can pray for your fellow group members on a regular basis. To whom will you send an email or write a card with the specific encouragement to reach his or her goals?

FAITH

- Put yourself aside and consider how you can plan a simple celebration for when a friend achieves a goal. Write down your plan below.

DAILY
CHECK-IN

FOOD

- How did your meals align with The Daniel Plan plate today?

- How would you rate your eating today on a scale of 1 to 10 (10 being best):

| 1 | 2 | 3 | 4 | 5 | 6 | 7 | 8 | 9 | 10 |

- Some of the best choices I made today were:
  (e.g., eating a healthy breakfast)

👟 FITNESS

- What type of fitness/movement did you do today?

- Duration:

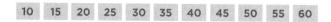

| 10 | 15 | 20 | 25 | 30 | 35 | 40 | 45 | 50 | 55 | 60 |

💡 FOCUS

- Gratitude for today:

- Goal for tomorrow:

👥 FRIENDS

- Who encouraged, supported, or joined you on your health journey today?

- Who needs your encouragement, support, or companionship?

DAILY
FOOD TRACKER

- What did you eat? How did it make you feel?

  BREAKFAST:

  SNACK:

  LUNCH:

  SNACK:

  DINNER:

  WATER: HOW MUCH WATER DID YOU DRINK?

- When you ate today, was it because you were hungry?
  Or were you motivated by boredom, stress, or fatigue?

- What worked?

- Any adjustments or changes for tomorrow?

10-Day Check-In

	DAY 30
Height	
Weight	
BMI*	
Blood Pressure	
Waist	
Hips	
Activity Level**	

*Refer to page 199 to calculate your BMI.
****Sedentary** (I rarely or never do any physical activities)
Light (I do some light or moderate physical activities every week)
Regular (I do moderate physical activities every week, 20–30 minutes a day for 3–4 days a week)
Active to vigorous (I do moderate to vigorous physical activities every week, 30–60 minutes a day for 5 or more days a week)

PERSONAL
ASSESSMENT

FAITH   **FOOD**   **FITNESS**   **FOCUS**   **FRIENDS**

- What Essentials have you been focusing on, and why?

- What progress have you made? *Celebrate your wins!*

- Is something still standing in your way? If so, what will you do differently to overcome it?

- What is something new you have learned about yourself?

- Based on what you have learned, what will you change next week?

- Already achieved your goals? *Congratulations!* It's time to set some new goals.

- Circle one to two *new* Essentials to focus on for the next ten days.

  FAITH   FOOD   FITNESS   FOCUS   FRIENDS

- Now set your SMART Goals, and share them with a friend!

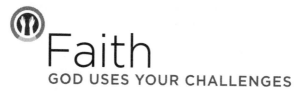

Faith

GOD USES YOUR CHALLENGES

As you received Christ Jesus the Lord, so continue to live in him. Keep your roots deep in him and have your lives built on him. Be strong in the faith.

— *Colossians 2:6 – 7 NCV*

DAILY
REFLECTION

It's easy to trust God when things are going great. But trust gets a little more challenging when things aren't going your way. God hears and answers every prayer you pray, but he doesn't always answer the way you want him to. Sometimes God says yes, sometimes no, and sometimes not yet. He may even say, "I have a different idea."

Trusting God even when you don't understand the way he answers your prayers becomes easier when you keep your roots deep in him. The way you respond to God's provision will build your faith as you trust in him.

🎯 FAITH

- Are you willing to trust God even when you don't get the answer you expected?

- What would your faith look like if you accepted that God uses challenges, including the ones you experience with your health, to help you mature and grow?

DAILY
CHECK-IN

🌀 FOOD

- How did your meals align with The Daniel Plan plate today?

- How would you rate your eating today on a scale of 1 to 10 (10 being best):

1   2   3   4   5   6   7   8   9   10

- Some of the best choices I made today were:
  (*e.g., eating a healthy breakfast*)

👟 FITNESS

- What type of fitness/movement did you do today?

- Duration:

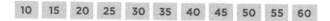

  10 15 20 25 30 35 40 45 50 55 60

💡 FOCUS

- Gratitude for today:

- Goal for tomorrow:

👥 FRIENDS

- Who encouraged, supported, or joined you on your health journey today?

- Who needs your encouragement, support, or companionship?

DAILY
FOOD TRACKER

- What did you eat? How did it make you feel?

  BREAKFAST:

  SNACK:

  LUNCH:

  SNACK:

  DINNER:

  WATER: HOW MUCH WATER DID YOU DRINK?

- When you ate today, was it because you were hungry? Or were you motivated by boredom, stress, or fatigue?

- What worked?

- Any adjustments or changes for tomorrow?

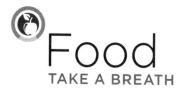

Food
TAKE A BREATH

We will never turn our back on you;
breathe life into our lungs so we can shout your name!
— *Psalm 80:18 MSG*

DAILY
REFLECTION

Breathing is one of the few functions of your body that you do automatically — but it can also be done mindfully. When you remember to breathe deeply, you can actually clear your body and mind. By slowing your breathing, you can lower your heart rate and your stress level. Breathing is a powerful way to strengthen your body.

Mindful breathing is a reminder to slow down and to think about our choices, whether with our faith, our food, our fitness, our focus, or our friends. For example, when we take a few deep breaths before we eat, we approach our eating more consciously. We eat less and enjoy it more.

Today, take some time to breathe slowly and deeply. God can breathe new life into you and your efforts to become healthier. "I will put breath in you, and you will come to life. Then you will know that I am the LORD" (Ezekiel 37:6).

Before your next meal, breathe in and out slowly a few times. How does it affect the way you eat and the way you feel during and after the meal?

FAITH

- What does it mean to "live and breathe God"? Why is this significant to your success in The Daniel Plan?

DAILY
CHECK-IN

FOOD

- How did your meals align with The Daniel Plan plate today?

- How would you rate your eating today on a scale of 1 to 10 (10 being best):

| 1 | 2 | 3 | 4 | 5 | 6 | 7 | 8 | 9 | 10 |

- Some of the best choices I made today were:
  (e.g., eating a healthy breakfast)

🏃 FITNESS

- What type of fitness/movement did you do today?

- Duration:

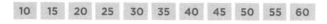

| 10 | 15 | 20 | 25 | 30 | 35 | 40 | 45 | 50 | 55 | 60 |

💡 FOCUS

- Gratitude for today:

- Goal for tomorrow:

👥 FRIENDS

- Who encouraged, supported, or joined you on your health journey today?

- Who needs your encouragement, support, or companionship?

DAILY
FOOD TRACKER

- What did you eat? How did it make you feel?

    BREAKFAST:

    SNACK:

    LUNCH:

    SNACK:

    DINNER:

    WATER: HOW MUCH WATER DID YOU DRINK?

- When you ate today, was it because you were hungry? Or were you motivated by boredom, stress, or fatigue?

- What worked?

- Any adjustments or changes for tomorrow?

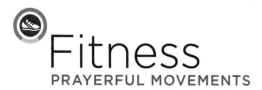

Fitness
PRAYERFUL MOVEMENTS

"He himself gives everyone life and breath and everything else.... God did this so that they would seek him and perhaps reach out for him and find him, though he is not far from any one of us. 'For in him we live and move and have our being'."

— Acts 17: 25, 27–28

DAILY
REFLECTION

The Daniel Plan integrates that which we tend to separate: faith, food, fitness, focus, and friends. Tackling the five Essentials together actually makes them easier.

In prayerful movements, our faith and fitness connect and strengthen one another, reminding us that in God "we live and move and have our being." He is the giver of life and breath.

When you take a walk, think of what it means to walk with God. When you get up to take a break from sitting, make a mental list of your blessings, or pray for the people in your home or workplace.

What do you notice about yourself as you engage in prayerful movement?

 FAITH

- Make a list of three prayerful movements that you will engage in today. There's no wrong way to do this — any movement is the right one!

DAILY
CHECK-IN

FOOD

- How did your meals align with The Daniel Plan plate today?

- How would you rate your eating today on a scale of 1 to 10 (10 being best):

| 1 | 2 | 3 | 4 | 5 | 6 | 7 | 8 | 9 | 10 |

- Some of the best choices I made today were:
  (e.g., eating a healthy breakfast)

👟 FITNESS

- What type of fitness/movement did you do today?

- Duration:

  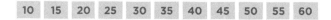

  | 10 | 15 | 20 | 25 | 30 | 35 | 40 | 45 | 50 | 55 | 60 |

💡 FOCUS

- Gratitude for today:

- Goal for tomorrow:

👥 FRIENDS

- Who encouraged, supported, or joined you on your
  health journey today?

- Who needs your encouragement, support, or
  companionship?

DAILY
FOOD TRACKER

- What did you eat? How did it make you feel?

  BREAKFAST:

  SNACK:

  LUNCH:

  SNACK:

  DINNER:

  WATER: HOW MUCH WATER DID YOU DRINK?

- When you ate today, was it because you were hungry?
  Or were you motivated by boredom, stress, or fatigue?

- What worked?

- Any adjustments or changes for tomorrow?

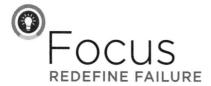

Focus
REDEFINE FAILURE

*The LORD directs the steps of the godly. He delights
in every detail of their lives. Though they stumble, they
will never fall, for the LORD holds them by the hand.*
— *Psalm 37:23–24 NLT*

DAILY
REFLECTION

The fear of failure is far more damaging than failure itself. Failing is not the end of the world. In fact, we vastly exaggerate the effects of failure.

How do you reduce that fear of failure? By redefining it. You haven't failed if you don't reach one of your Daniel Plan goals. On The Daniel Plan you cannot fail, because there is no end date. If you have a setback, overdo it on a dessert, or miss an opportunity to move your body, tomorrow is a new day. Setbacks are simply part of the journey that you use to learn and grow.

Consider that every "mistake" teaches you a way that won't work and takes you closer to discovering what will work. Mistakes also remind us that we need God's help, which builds our faith. When we admit our weakness, God shows up and strengthens us.

🎭 FAITH

- What would your journey toward a healthier life look like if you went through each day depending on Jesus?

- What can you learn from your failures or mistakes? How can they move you forward instead of setting you back?

DAILY
CHECK-IN

FOOD

- How did your meals align with The Daniel Plan plate today?

- How would you rate your eating today on a scale of 1 to 10 (10 being best):

  | 1 | 2 | 3 | 4 | 5 | 6 | 7 | 8 | 9 | 10 |

- Some of the best choices I made today were:
  (e.g., eating a healthy breakfast)

FITNESS

- What type of fitness/movement did you do today?

- Duration:

  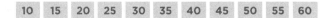

FOCUS

- Gratitude for today:

- Goal for tomorrow:

FRIENDS

- Who encouraged, supported, or joined you on your health journey today?

- Who needs your encouragement, support, or companionship?

DAILY
FOOD TRACKER

- What did you eat? How did it make you feel?

  BREAKFAST:

  SNACK:

  LUNCH:

  SNACK:

  DINNER:

  WATER: HOW MUCH WATER DID YOU DRINK?

- When you ate today, was it because you were hungry?
  Or were you motivated by boredom, stress, or fatigue?

- What worked?

- Any adjustments or changes for tomorrow?

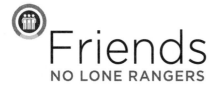

Friends
NO LONE RANGERS

A person standing alone can be attacked and defeated, but two can stand back-to-back and conquer. Three are even better, for a triple-braided cord is not easily broken.
— Ecclesiastes 4:12 NLT

DAILY
REFLECTION

There are some things in your life that you will never be able to change without the support, prayers, and encouragement of other people. Success takes teamwork.

Even Jesus didn't go it alone. He had a circle of twelve friends and three close buddies. Plus, he talked to his Father all the time. In order to find long-lasting health and strength, you absolutely need a small group of friends to support you.

On your own, you are more likely to get discouraged and give up when challenges come. But working together, you can encourage one another to keep going when the journey gets tough.

What are some things you feel discouraged about? Share those things with your group.

FAITH

- If you are resistant to receiving help or support, why do you think that's so? Ask God to show you why, and ask him to prepare you to receive help.

- Proverbs 27:17 says, "As iron sharpens iron, so one person sharpens another." How do your closest friends sharpen you intellectually? How do they encourage you to grow?

DAILY
CHECK-IN

FOOD

- How did your meals align with The Daniel Plan plate today?

- How would you rate your eating today on a scale of 1 to 10 (10 being best):

1   2   3   4   5   6   7   8   9   10

- Some of the best choices I made today were:
  (e.g., eating a healthy breakfast)

👟 FITNESS

- What type of fitness/movement did you do today?

- Duration:

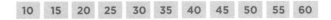

💡 FOCUS

- Gratitude for today:

- Goal for tomorrow:

👥 FRIENDS

- Who encouraged, supported, or joined you on your health journey today?

- Who needs your encouragement, support, or companionship?

DAILY
FOOD TRACKER

- What did you eat? How did it make you feel?

  BREAKFAST:

  SNACK:

  LUNCH:

  SNACK:

  DINNER:

  WATER: HOW MUCH WATER DID YOU DRINK?

- When you ate today, was it because you were hungry? Or were you motivated by boredom, stress, or fatigue?

- What worked?

- Any adjustments or changes for tomorrow?

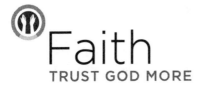

Faith
TRUST GOD MORE

[Jesus] said, "Come ahead." Jumping out of the boat, Peter walked on the water to Jesus. But when he looked down at the waves churning beneath his feet, he lost his nerve and started to sink. He cried, "Master, save me!" Jesus didn't hesitate. He reached down and grabbed his hand. Then he said, "Faint-heart, what got into you?"

— Matthew 14:29–31 MSG

DAILY
REFLECTION

Most of the time when we say we need more faith, we think that means we have to *try* harder to trust God. But the truth is, our faith increases when we take tangible steps toward trusting God.

Peter's faith increased when he stepped out of the boat. Without that step, he wouldn't have been able to see that Jesus was going to help him walk on the water. But when Peter looked at the waves around him, he lost his focus on Jesus and immediately began to sink.

The Bible says Jesus didn't hesitate to reach out and save Peter. Then he gave Peter a gentle rebuke — no condemnation, just a question to help Peter think about how to keep his eyes on Jesus.

🎭 FAITH

- What are some areas of The Daniel Plan in which you have been working harder but really just need to trust God more?

- How and where have you seen God increase your faith to help you become healthier in your faith, body, or mind?

DAILY
CHECK-IN

🍴 FOOD

- How did your meals align with The Daniel Plan plate today?

- How would you rate your eating today on a scale of 1 to 10 (10 being best):

| 1 | 2 | 3 | 4 | 5 | 6 | 7 | 8 | 9 | 10 |

- Some of the best choices I made today were:
  (e.g., eating a healthy breakfast)

👟 FITNESS

- What type of fitness/movement did you do today?

- Duration:

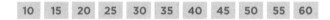

| 10 | 15 | 20 | 25 | 30 | 35 | 40 | 45 | 50 | 55 | 60 |

💡 FOCUS

- Gratitude for today:

- Goal for tomorrow:

👥 FRIENDS

- Who encouraged, supported, or joined you on your health journey today?

- Who needs your encouragement, support, or companionship?

DAILY
FOOD TRACKER

- What did you eat? How did it make you feel?

  BREAKFAST:

  SNACK:

  LUNCH:

  SNACK:

  DINNER:

  WATER: HOW MUCH WATER DID YOU DRINK?

- When you ate today, was it because you were hungry? Or were you motivated by boredom, stress, or fatigue?

- What worked?

- Any adjustments or changes for tomorrow?

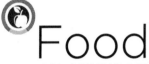Food

AN ABUNDANCE OF THE BEST

But Jesus said, "There is no need to dismiss them. You give them supper."

"All we have are five loaves of bread and two fish," they said.

Jesus said, "Bring them here." Then he had the people sit on the grass. He took the five loaves and two fish, lifted his face to heaven in prayer, blessed, broke, and gave the bread to the disciples. The disciples then gave the food to the congregation. They all ate their fill. They gathered twelve baskets of leftovers.

— Matthew 14:16 – 20 MSG

DAILY
REFLECTION

You don't have to worry about your next meal, because God knows what you need and has promised to take care of you. He also knows what your body needs to function well. The food that he wants to give you in great supply is the food that is best for your body.

The Daniel Plan is not about deprivation. God has provided you with an abundance of good food: fresh vegetables, seeds, nuts, fruits, legumes, and meats. You can eat plenty of these foods in The Daniel Plan, and the nutrients they provide will strengthen you.

As you learn about the power of eating God's best, food doesn't have to be harmful but medicine that heals and nourishes your body.

🍎 FAITH

- In what ways has food become more important to you than feeding on God's Word?

- Why do you think eating the right food requires faith?

DAILY
CHECK-IN

🍎 FOOD

- How did your meals align with The Daniel Plan plate today?

- How would you rate your eating today on a scale of 1 to 10 (10 being best):

| 1 | 2 | 3 | 4 | 5 | 6 | 7 | 8 | 9 | 10 |

- Some of the best choices I made today were:
  (e.g., eating a healthy breakfast)

● FITNESS

- What type of fitness/movement did you do today?

- Duration:

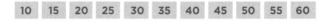

● FOCUS

- Gratitude for today:

- Goal for tomorrow:

● FRIENDS

- Who encouraged, supported, or joined you on your health journey today?

- Who needs your encouragement, support, or companionship?

DAILY
FOOD TRACKER

- What did you eat? How did it make you feel?

   BREAKFAST:

   SNACK:

   LUNCH:

   SNACK:

   DINNER:

   WATER: HOW MUCH WATER DID YOU DRINK?

- When you ate today, was it because you were hungry? Or were you motivated by boredom, stress, or fatigue?

- What worked?

- Any adjustments or changes for tomorrow?

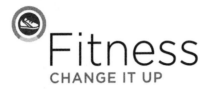
Fitness
CHANGE IT UP

O Lord, what a variety of things you have made!
In wisdom you have made them all.
The earth is full of your creatures.
— *Psalm 104:24 NLT*

DAILY
REFLECTION

Look around and you can see that God loves variety. He created people in different shapes and sizes. There are all kinds of trees and plants and so many choices for things we can eat. We even have choices within choices. For example, there are more than 7,500 varieties of apples.

God knows we need change and variety, and that includes our exercise routine. If your routine falls into a rut, exercise becomes less effective, and boredom (or even burnout) can creep in. That's why mixing it up can add new life to your fitness experience. You might get creative with your cardio and wacky with your weight training.

Changing your routine not only boosts your fitness, but can sharpen your focus as well. Driving a different route to work, trying a new kind of food, learning a new skill, or even meeting new people can help your brain and body stay healthy and active.

What can keep you from getting bored with fitness?

FAITH

- How can you change your routine — in fitness, food, and faith practices — so that your energy and focus are renewed?

DAILY
CHECK-IN

FOOD

- How did your meals align with The Daniel Plan plate today?

- How would you rate your eating today on a scale of 1 to 10 (10 being best):

| 1 | 2 | 3 | 4 | 5 | 6 | 7 | 8 | 9 | 10 |

- Some of the best choices I made today were:
  (e.g., eating a healthy breakfast)

🏃 FITNESS

- What type of fitness/movement did you do today?

- Duration:

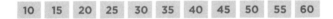

💡 FOCUS

- Gratitude for today:

- Goal for tomorrow:

👥 FRIENDS

- Who encouraged, supported, or joined you on your health journey today?

- Who needs your encouragement, support, or companionship?

DAILY
FOOD TRACKER

- What did you eat? How did it make you feel?

  BREAKFAST:

  SNACK:

  LUNCH:

  SNACK:

  DINNER:

  WATER: HOW MUCH WATER DID YOU DRINK?

- When you ate today, was it because you were hungry?
  Or were you motivated by boredom, stress, or fatigue?

- What worked?

- Any adjustments or changes for tomorrow?

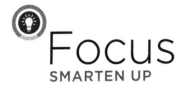

Focus
SMARTEN UP

*Give careful thought to the paths for your feet
and be steadfast in all your ways.*
— *Proverbs 4:26*

DAILY
REFLECTION

Setting goals is not just a good idea, but also a spiritual discipline. Goals stretch you and help you become all God wants you to be.

God is a God who sets goals, and he expects you to set them, too. As suggested earlier, setting goals will give a destination for your vision. Move forward toward health in all areas of life, and accomplish what God has called you to do by revisiting your SMART Goals. They will set you up for long-lasting change.

FAITH

- Start thinking and praying about the SMART Goals you can set for the next forty days. What is God prompting you to aim for? Ask God to show you the steps to get there.

- How do your goals reflect a desire to grow in Christ-likeness and bring glory to God?

DAILY
CHECK-IN

FOOD

- How did your meals align with The Daniel Plan plate today?

- How would you rate your eating today on a scale of 1 to 10 (10 being best):

| 1 | 2 | 3 | 4 | 5 | 6 | 7 | 8 | 9 | 10 |

- Some of the best choices I made today were:
  (e.g., eating a healthy breakfast)

🏃 FITNESS

- What type of fitness/movement did you do today?

- Duration:

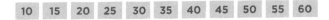

💡 FOCUS

- Gratitude for today:

- Goal for tomorrow:

👥 FRIENDS

- Who encouraged, supported, or joined you on your health journey today?

- Who needs your encouragement, support, or companionship?

DAILY
FOOD TRACKER

- What did you eat? How did it make you feel?

   BREAKFAST:

   SNACK:

   LUNCH:

   SNACK:

   DINNER:

   WATER: HOW MUCH WATER DID YOU DRINK?

- When you ate today, was it because you were hungry? Or were you motivated by boredom, stress, or fatigue?

- What worked?

- Any adjustments or changes for tomorrow?

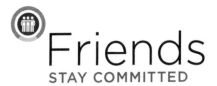

Friends
STAY COMMITTED

*You can develop a healthy, robust community that lives right with God and enjoy its results **only** if you do the hard work of getting along with each other, treating each other with dignity and honor.*

— James 3:18 MSG

DAILY
REFLECTION

For you to become healthy for life, you need to be committed to a small group of friends who will love and support you in your Daniel Plan journey and for the rest of your life.

Your friends need the same commitment from you. The Daniel Plan is not just for forty days, but for a lifetime of pursuing God's best for your health — spiritually, emotionally, and physically.

Commit to loving each other even at your worst, when you want to unload your frustrations, and when you have slipped up on The Daniel Plan four weeks in a row. Commit to loving each other as Christ loved you. Commit to carrying each other's burdens and helping each other beyond these first forty days toward better health. Set new goals with a few friends or your group, and continue moving forward.

Whom do you know who is committed to you and your success? As you conclude this forty-day journey, what could you do to make that a long-lasting friendship?

FAITH

- With which friends or group members can you renew your commitment for faith, health, and the next steps of your Daniel Plan journey?

DAILY
CHECK-IN

FOOD

- How did your meals align with The Daniel Plan plate today?

- How would you rate your eating today on a scale of 1 to 10 (10 being best):

| 1 | 2 | 3 | 4 | 5 | 6 | 7 | 8 | 9 | 10 |

- Some of the best choices I made today were:
  (e.g., eating a healthy breakfast)

🏃 FITNESS

- What type of fitness/movement did you do today?

- Duration:

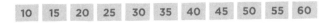

💡 FOCUS

- Gratitude for today:

- Goal for tomorrow:

👥 FRIENDS

- Who encouraged, supported, or joined you on your health journey today?

- Who needs your encouragement, support, or companionship?

DAILY
FOOD TRACKER

- What did you eat? How did it make you feel?

  BREAKFAST:

  SNACK:

  LUNCH:

  SNACK:

  DINNER:

  WATER: HOW MUCH WATER DID YOU DRINK?

- When you ate today, was it because you were hungry? Or were you motivated by boredom, stress, or fatigue?

- What worked?

- Any adjustments or changes for tomorrow?

40-Day Health Assessment

Re-record your numbers from DAY 1	
Height	
Weight	
BMI*	
Blood Pressure	
Waist	
Hips	
Activity Level**	

DAY 40	
Height	
Weight	
BMI*	
Blood Pressure	
Waist	
Hips	
Activity Level**	

*Refer to page 199 to calculate your BMI.

**Sedentary (I rarely or never do any physical activities)
Light (I do some light or moderate physical activities every week)
Regular (I do moderate physical activities every week, 20–30 minutes a day for 3–4 days a week)
Active to vigorous (I do moderate to vigorous physical activities every week, 30–60 minutes a day for 5 or more days a week)

PERSONAL
ASSESSMENT

 FAITH

 FOOD

 FITNESS

 FOCUS

 FRIENDS

- What Essentials did you focus on over the past forty days?

- What progress did you make? *Celebrate your wins!*

- Is something still standing in your way? If so, what will you do differently to overcome it?

- What is something new you have learned about yourself?

- Based on what you've learned, what will you change up moving forward?

Next Steps

Now that you have lived out your Daniel Plan experience for the past forty days, how do you feel? You have likely made progress, and it is likely that the changes are becoming part of your everyday lifestyle. Congratulations! This is your new normal.

Here's the great news: This is just the beginning! The Daniel Plan 40-Day Journal experience is designed to *launch* you on your journey to health. During these forty days we have equipped you with spiritual inspiration and the basics of the five Essentials. The momentum from taking your early small steps is starting to take hold.

As you have learned, tracking your progress is key to sustaining change. Here are more practical next steps to choose from as you continue your journey to a healthier life!

Continue journaling: Get a new blank journal, create your own, or check out The Daniel Plan App (available at *danielplan. com*) to track your progress and connect with other people.

Set up your FREE health profile: If you haven't already done so, go to *danielplan.com* and set up your FREE health profile today.

Sign up for our weekly newsletter: Sign up at *danielplan.com* to receive our weekly recipes, practical resources, everyday encouragement, biblical inspiration, fitness tips, and more.

Create new SMART Goals in faith: Now that you have experienced the thrill of achieving your goals, it's time to take your health to a new level — think big!

Lead a new small-group study: Invite some friends to start a new small group. Go through *The Daniel Plan* six-session video-based study together. This study will teach you the foundational principles of The Daniel Plan, with biblical inspiration from Pastor Warren, our founding doctors, and our wellness experts. Learn more at *danielplan.com.*

Share The Daniel Plan: Now that you have a taste of everything The Daniel Plan has to offer, why not share it with a friend, co-worker, or neighbor? Tell your faith community about it. Give the gift of health today.

BMI Chart

BMI	HEALTHY WEIGHT						OVERWEIGHT				
	19	20	21	22	23	24	25	26	27	28	29
Height	Body Weight in Pounds										
4'10"	91	96	100	105	110	115	119	124	129	134	138
4'11"	94	99	104	109	114	119	124	128	133	138	143
5'	97	102	107	112	118	123	128	133	138	143	148
5'1"	100	106	111	116	122	127	132	137	143	148	153
5'2"	104	109	115	120	126	131	136	142	147	153	158
5'3"	107	113	118	124	130	135	141	146	152	158	163
5'4"	110	116	122	128	134	140	145	151	157	163	169
5'5"	114	120	126	132	138	144	150	156	162	168	174
5'6"	118	124	130	136	142	148	155	161	167	173	179
5'7"	121	127	134	140	146	153	159	166	172	178	185
5'8"	125	131	138	144	151	158	164	171	177	184	190
5'9"	128	135	142	149	155	162	169	176	182	189	196
5'10"	132	139	146	153	160	167	174	181	188	195	202
5'11"	136	143	150	157	165	172	179	186	193	200	208
6'	140	147	154	162	169	177	184	191	199	206	213
6'1"	144	151	159	166	174	182	189	197	204	212	219
6'2"	148	155	163	171	179	186	194	202	210	218	225
6'3"	152	160	168	176	184	192	200	208	216	224	232
6'4"	156	164	172	180	189	197	205	213	221	230	238

BMI CHART cont.

BMI	30	31	32	33	34	35	36	37	38	39	40
						OBESE					
Height					Body Weight in Pounds						
4'10"	143	148	153	158	162	167	172	177	181	186	191
4'11"	148	153	158	163	168	173	178	183	188	193	198
5'	153	158	163	168	174	179	184	189	194	199	204
5'1"	158	164	169	174	180	185	190	195	201	206	211
5'2"	164	169	175	180	186	191	196	202	207	213	218
5'3"	169	175	180	186	191	197	203	208	214	220	225
5'4"	174	180	186	192	197	204	209	215	221	227	232
5'5"	180	186	192	198	204	210	216	222	228	234	240
5'6"	186	192	198	204	210	216	223	229	235	241	247
5'7"	191	198	204	211	217	223	230	236	242	249	255
5'8"	197	203	210	216	223	230	236	243	249	256	262
5'9"	203	209	216	223	230	236	243	250	257	263	270
5'10"	209	216	222	229	236	243	250	257	264	271	278
5'11"	215	222	229	236	243	250	257	265	272	279	286
6'	221	228	235	242	250	258	265	272	279	287	294
6'1"	227	235	242	250	257	265	272	280	288	295	302
6'2"	233	241	249	256	264	272	280	287	295	303	311
6'3"	240	248	256	264	272	279	287	295	303	311	319
6'4"	246	254	263	271	279	287	295	304	312	320	328

Contributors

Dee Eastman is the director of The Daniel Plan at Saddleback Church and has a passion for helping people move their way to better health while drawing closer to God. Dee is an active speaker and co-authored a Bible study curriculum that has sold more than 3 million copies.

Jon Walker, managing editor of Rick Warren's Daily Hope Devotionals, is a pastor, writer, and editor who has served the Saddleback Church community in communications for almost fifteen years. He is also the founding editor of Rick Warren's Ministry ToolBox.

Keri Wyatt Kent, author and speaker, is a regular contributor to several magazines, websites, and blogs. She has written ten books and co-authored several others.

Sean Foy, president and founder of the Personal Wellness Corporation, is an exercise physiologist, behavioral coach, and speaker. He is also the author and developer of the signature fitness program for The Biggest Loser Pro Training program.

April O'Neil, writer and communications specialist for The Daniel Plan, is also a certified holistic health coach and founder of Nourished Women. Her passion is to teach people how to heal physically, spiritually, and emotionally.

Shelly Antol, operations and marketing manager for The Daniel Plan, manages key projects such as *The Daniel Plan Cookbook*. She has been a community leader for women's small groups and led the MOPS Ministry at Saddleback Church.

Kathrine Lee, co-creator and executive director of The Ultimate Source, is an internationally recognized speaker and has touched millions with her message of hope and transformation. Kathrine is a member of The Daniel Plan Board of Advisors.

Brian Williams, author, board certified life coach, and ordained pastor, has extensive experience helping people create life transformation. Using accountability and encouragement, he has an individualized approach that helps people succeed to achieve their goals.

THE **DANIEL** PLAN

The Daniel Plan
40 Days to a Healthier Life

*Rick Warren D.Min.,
Daniel Amen M.D.,
and Mark Hyman M.D.*

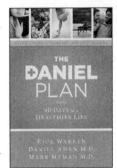

The Daniel Plan: 40 Days to a Healthier Life by Rick Warren, Dr. Daniel Amen, and Dr. Mark Hyman is an innovative approach to achieving a healthy lifestyle where people get better together by optimizing their health in the key life areas of faith, food, fitness, focus, and friends. Within these five key life Essentials, readers are offered a multitude of resources and the foundation to get healthy. Ultimately, *The Daniel Plan* is about abundance, not deprivation, and this is why the plan is both transformational and sustainable. *The Daniel Plan* teaches simple ways to incorporate healthy choices into your current lifestyle, while encouraging you to rely on God's power through biblical principles. Readers are encouraged to do The Daniel Plan with another person or a group to maximize their potential to experience an all-around healthy lifestyle. Readers are offered cutting-edge, real-world applications that are easy to implement and create tangible results.

Available in stores and online!

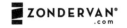

The Daniel Plan Cookbook

Healthy Eating for Life

Rick Warren D.Min.,
Daniel Amen M.D.,
and Mark Hyman M.D.

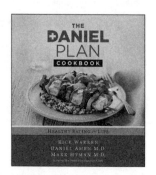

The Daniel Plan Cookbook: Healthy Cooking for Life is a four-color cookbook filled with 100 delicious, Daniel Plan–approved recipes that offer an abundance of options to bring healthy cooking back into your kitchen. This eye-appealing cookbook is filled with easy-to-prepare, mouth-watering recipes. All the recipes are based on The Daniel Plan plate that emphasizes eating nutritionally packed whole foods. Choose from a variety of delicious options to create your weekly menu. Eating The Daniel Plan way not only is healthy and wholesome, but will boost your energy and kick-start your metabolism. The book includes practical tips from doctors, important food facts, and inspiration from the Daniel Plan signature chefs.

Available in stores and online!

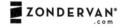
ZONDERVAN
.com

The Daniel Plan Mobile APP

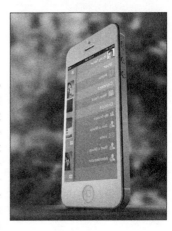

The healthy Daniel Plan App will be a dynamic app based on the cookbook/fitness book content but in a succinct, easy-to-understand-and-use format that provides wisdom and encouragement for each interaction. App will include a calorie counter, a feature for tracking progress on weight loss and improving BMI (including the formula for calculating BMI), as well as a simple exercise log. Encouragement coupled with dietary facts and/or recipe ideas can be pushed to the user.

Available in stores and online!

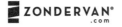

Share Your Thoughts

Free Online Resources at
www.zondervan.com

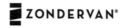